P9-CLE-725

UNDERSTANDING CHILDHOOD HEARING LOSS

Whole Family Approaches to Living and Thriving

Brian J. Fligor

ROWMAN & LITTLEFIELD
Lanham • Boulder • New York • London

Published by Rowman & Littlefield
A wholly owned subsidiary of The Rowman & Littlefield Publishing Group, Inc.
4501 Forbes Boulevard, Suite 200, Lanham, Maryland 20706
www.rowman.com

Unit A, Whitacre Mews, 26-34 Stannary Street, London SE11 4AB

British Library Cataloguing in Publication Information Available

Library of Congress Cataloging-in-Publication Data

Fligor, Brian J.
Understanding childhood hearing loss: Whole family approaches to living and thriving / by Brian J. Fligor.
p. cm. (Whole family approaches to childhood illness and disorders)
Includes bibliographical references and index.
ISBN 978-1-4422-2666-1 (cloth : alk. paper) -- ISBN 978-1-4422-2667-8 (electronic)
I. Title. II. Series: Whole family approaches to childhood illness and disorders.
[DNLM: 1. Child. 2. Hearing Loss. 3. Family--psychology. 4. Infant. 5. Self Help Groups. 6. Social Support. WV 270]
RF290 2015
617.80083--dc23
2015013359

Printed in the United States of America

CONTENTS

ACKNOWLEDGMENTS

I wish to thank my family for their undying support through many hours of my absence as I wrote this book. Huge thanks go to my wife, Jana, for always having my back, managing a house full of young children with minimal backup, and instilling our home with lots of laughter and fun. My unconditional love to Kensie, Emma, Josh, and Danielle, for calling me "Rabbit" instead of "Daddy" and for teaching me more about child development than I could have ever learned in university training. My heartfelt thanks to my mentors, in particular Clarke Cox, Maryellen Curran, David Citron, and Marilyn Neault, for pushing me to my potential. My deep appreciation to my friend and colleague Lydia Gregoret for her review of chapter 5, "How Hearing Loss Is Treated," and for sharing her stories of her family's experience raising a son with hearing loss. And finally, my deep gratitude to my patients and their families, for allowing me to become part of your lives, for letting me be with you to share in difficult conversations, and proving to me how resilient families can be.

WELCOME TO HOLLAND . . . A CLINICIAN'S PERSPECTIVE

Emily Perl Kingsley wrote an essay in 1987 entitled "Welcome to Holland."[1] As a mother of a child with developmental challenges, Ms. Kingsley penned the essay as a way to describe what it is like to be surprised by the life-altering event of becoming a parent of a child with special developmental needs. In the essay, she uses a vacation to Italy as a metaphor to describe the typical, lovely, romantic notion of what delightful experiences parenthood will bring. The excitement, the planning, the travel guides, and so on are all about the sights and sounds of Italy. When the day arrives for the giddy parents to fly to "Italy," the plane instead lands in Holland. And there are no flights to Italy; Holland is where these new parents will stay, despite the fact that they are not familiar with the territory, language, challenges, or delights. After the initial shock, the essay builds a sense of hope that there are new and beautiful things in Holland; however, there is a clear thread of the parents going through the stages of grief (from denial to acceptance) and a lasting sense of longing for Italy in this brief and poignant essay.

When I was in my final year of clinical training as an audiologist at Boston Children's Hospital, my fellow trainees and I were given "Welcome to Holland." Our clinical instructors intended to help us inexperienced, but well-intentioned, clinicians-in-training consider the perspective of the parents of children we served. I was not a parent at the time, and had been relatively untouched personally by significant medical or developmental needs in children. My own education in participating in the care for these perfect children was a steep learning curve, and my education will continue until the day I can no longer provide direct clinical service. When that happens, I hope I have the opportunity to continue to teach students and junior audiologists in welcoming new parents to "Holland."

Now, speaking from the experience of having four children (three girls and one boy, ages six months through seven years old, at the time of writing), parenthood is not a vacation. My children are medically and developmentally typical, and I can think of no other experience harder, more frustrating, expensive, heartbreaking, and joyous. Before my first child was born, I foolishly thought "I've had to pull all-nighters before in college. I'm sure I'll manage a sleepless newborn just fine." Parents reading this are surely laughing right along with me now. I do not know what it is like to be a parent who is told "I'm glad we were able to get a great test on your baby today, because were learned something very important about his/her hearing." But I am a parent who has said those words to new parents perhaps a couple hundred times in the last decade.

Since nearly all babies have their hearing screened in the hospital shortly after they are born and before they go home for the first time, children born with hearing loss often have their first hearing test when they are very young; perhaps as young as only a couple weeks old. When state-coordinated newborn hearing screening programs are working as they are intended (with a goal of early diagnosis of and intervention for hearing loss), the diagnosis of hearing loss is driven by the medical community, not by the parents. While early diagnosis and intervention does result in better outcomes for a child's speech and language development (all things being equal), it creates significant challenges for the parents that might be (and often are) overlooked by the well-intentioned clinicians.[2] Prior to the technology existing that allows us to screen newborns for hearing loss, parents of children with suspected hearing loss were challenged to find their way to a pediatric-specialized audiologist to determine if the child did, or did not, have hearing loss. The parents were almost universally the ones who first suspected the hearing loss, either through observation of lack of awareness of certain sounds (sometimes they only seemed to miss soft sounds, sometimes they seemed to miss all sounds, no matter how loud) or lack of making good progress in learning to talk. The suspicions for hearing loss would often be brought first to the child's family doctor or pediatrician, who may or may not immediately send the family to another specialist (an audiologist or ear, nose, and throat physician).[3] If the primary care doctor took a conservative approach ("watchful waiting"), often times the child with speech-delay would catch up to peers, or at least make good progress on his or her own. "Watchful waiting" for speech-delay means observing if the child starts making good progress in spoken language acquisition without "overdoing it" by ordering potentially unnecessary tests. If parents were adamant their child must be seen for a hearing test, this testing was usually months after suspicions for hearing loss first arose. In those children who did have hearing loss, parents' suspicions were validated, and parents were primed to advocate for their child's newly discovered developmental needs.

When a baby doesn't pass the hearing screening in the hospital and an appointment has been made for follow-up testing with an audiologist, there is seldom any reason for parents to have suspicion their baby has a hearing loss. Therefore, instead of parents driving the effort to find out how good is their baby's hearing, the medical community is driving the effort. In preparation for the formal hearing test that is done if a baby doesn't pass the newborn hearing screening in the hospital, the parents are often told "bring the baby hungry and tired but not yet asleep." The reason for these instructions is newborns cannot reliably show how good their hearing is through their behavior. That is, newborns don't *reliably* turn their head to sound, or startle to sounds they hear, or otherwise make obvious by their behavior if their hearing is good enough to hear all the sounds of speech, which is fundamental to the child learning how to talk and to refine their language skills over the next several years. Instead, the audiologist performs tests that measure ear and nerve responses ("objective" tests) when playing sounds to the baby's ears. The responses that come from the ear and nerves are very small, and can only be recorded with specialized equipment in very quiet rooms. If the baby is moving, the responses typically cannot be recorded, and the hearing test is inconclusive. If the baby is crying, testing is not possible. So, bringing the baby hungry and tired, but not yet asleep means greatest likelihood of the baby falling asleep quickly and staying asleep for the forty-five to ninety minutes it takes to do the "sleep hearing tests." But that means the sleep-deprived, postpartum parents come to the appointment already at their wits' end. Their baby may have been crying the entire trip to the hospital, may have spit-up on the car seat, herself, and her parent. The parents might be struggling with breastfeeding. They might be struggling with finances. They might be arguing more than they have ever in their entire relationship. And they may be given news that changes their lives.

Diagnosing a hearing loss may be more of a process than an event. If testing runs very efficiently (the baby remains quietly sleeping the entire appointment; all the test results make sense and don't contradict one another; etc.), a fairly complete picture of the hearing loss can be defined in that one test. However, during the forty-five to ninety minutes of testing, the audiologist is uncovering new information about the baby's hearing in bits and pieces. It is somewhat like putting together a jigsaw puzzle, where pieces match together to show an overall picture. When the picture is complete (or the baby wakes and testing has to be ended), the audiologist describes the picture to the parents and uses this information to recommend next steps. If the picture is not complete enough to direct recommendations, repeat testing is necessary to fill in "puzzle pieces."

While the audiologist is putting together the puzzle pieces during the testing, parents do not know what picture is developing. But the audiologist does. The difference in knowledge can create a tension between the parents and the clinician, as the audiologist begins to know more about the baby's hearing than the parents. This gives the audiologist time to develop his or her recommendations, and how to approach the (likely difficult) conversation with the parents; it also gives the audiologist time to become anxious about how good, or bad, this difficult conversation might go. Clinicians are typically empathic people, striving to heal pain. While the audiologist is uncovering a new hearing loss, they are anticipating providing valuable information that will almost always be painful for the family to hear. It is also painful to deliver. And the anticipation of delivering painful news can often be misinterpreted by the audiologist as believing he or she is "causing" the pain.

A DIFFICULT CONVERSATION

For sake of illustrating a hypothetical exchange between a parent of a child newly diagnosed with hearing loss and the audiologist, the following vignette is offered. This is an example of what can be called a "difficult conversation" between the audiologist and parent, and is meant to be considered from the parent's perspective. It does not recount any particular exchange between a parent and the audiologist, but draws from several similar scenarios I witnessed, or where I was the audiologist, and is informed by conversations with several parents describing for me their experience with learning their child had permanent hearing loss. It is neither perfectly delivered, nor perfectly flawed, but is an attempt at showing how this conversation is a mix of good intent and a delivery that is, at best, modestly successful. Some go better than this, some go worse. This hypothetical exchange is also very brief, relative to how these conversations usually go. In parentheses are hypothetical examples of the parent's observations of the audiologist's behavior, or about the environment, which are oddly present to the parent in this instance:

> Audiologist (projecting confidence): "Your baby slept beautifully through the whole test and we got all the information we could have wanted. We now know that he has hearing loss, and it's the kind of hearing loss that can't be cured with medicine or surgery."

Parent (the words haven't hit yet; it's like a split second calm before a train collision): "But they told me in the hospital I shouldn't worry, that he failed the screening because there was fluid in his ears."

Audiologist (using a soft, kind voice): "We know from some of the tests we did today that there isn't any fluid in the ears, but his hearing is in the mild-to-moderate hearing loss range. This means he can hear some louder sounds, especially when he's close by. There are a lot of speech sounds, though, that he can't hear."

Parent (tears are welling up, or falling, with a sense of panic setting in): "But that means he can hear something, right? Can he have some kind of therapy to help him hear better?"

Audiologist (adjusts in the chair, she is wearing a sweater. The pattern of the sweater is nothing I would ever wear, but is a good color for the audiologist): "We can help your baby hear better by fitting him with hearing aids, and getting him into early intervention with a speech-language pathologist to help him use his hearing with hearing aids to learn to talk."

Parent (full panic): "You mean he might not learn how to talk?"

Audiologist (stops breathing, why did she stop breathing? Is it that bad!?): "He *should*. But he needs hearing aids and speech therapy, and it's going to take a lot of work."

Parent (looks back and forth around the room; why are we in such a small room? Don't they have bigger rooms? The walls look so close, it seems like they are closing in, and it's hard to breathe in here): "What if he just wears one hearing aid, will that be enough?"

Audiologist (shifts again, I heard a sigh. Why did she sigh? I can tell she sighed. Does she think I said something stupid?): "We'll figure out what we need to do as we go along. What's important now is we know this information and we have a good idea what to do about it.

I'm going to give you a folder with information about services for children with hearing loss, so you can look at it when you are ready."

Parent (now my ears aren't working, I don't understand what's being said. I need to pay attention but I can't. I feel so lost and hopeless!): "What could have caused this?"

Audiologist (leaning forward . . . good, I asked a question she knows the answer to, she seems to project confidence again): "Blah, blah, genetics, blah . . . infections, blah . . . have him seen by an ENT, blah . . ."

Parent (looking back and forth, as though seeking an exit . . . thinking, "I swear she spoke English but I didn't understand a word she said. What's wrong with *my* ears?!"): "Can he just wear one hearing aid?"

Audiologist (she sat back again and shifted. Her chin raised a little. She doesn't like the question I just asked): "Since he has hearing loss in both ears, it would be best for him to use two."

Parent (melting back into the chair, shoulders slumping; thinking, "I know that, I know that, of course, if there's two ears that don't hear well we need two hearing aids. Why did I ask that?"): "You have a folder for me?"

Audiologist (she leaned forward again. Ok, this is something she can do. She can't do much, can she? Wow, I shouldn't have thought that, she's only trying to help. Can I get out of here?): "Yes, this folder has information blah, blah . . . the Department of blah blah blah. . . . And we can blah, jargon jargon . . ."

Parent: (Quiet)

Of course, this is just an example of a difficult conversation. Many do have an exchange like this, and many are different: both better, and worse. But time and again, in recalling the experience of having been told that their child has hearing loss, parents recount that they heard only the first five minutes (maybe) of the conversation, but the "counseling" lasted much longer than that. In the example above, the parent exhibits, in words, behaviors, and thoughts, normal reactions to a highly abnormal situation. Being told your child has permanent hearing loss is not a normal situation. And so to protect oneself from the pain, the parent in this example tries briefly to deny the loss ("but they told me it was just fluid"), bargaining ("Can he just wear one hearing aid?"), as well as typical fight-or-flight reactions (the walls are closing in, I can't breathe, I'm noticing *everything* in this room as though knowing these trivial pieces of information is life or death, I need to leave). And while in this example the audiologist provided an appropriately modest amount of excellent information and communicated that information with empathy, the audiologist made a common mistake: very often, questions parents ask in this situation are masked as "information" questions when in fact they are "affective" questions. "Affective" questions are ones that reflect the parent's need for the audiologist to recognize and witness the pain the parent is feeling, in a nonjudgmental way. Parents usually do not feel they have permission to react with grief, or they simply want to avoid these feelings at all costs, and so mask their request for permission by phrasing their affective questions as ones seeking factual information. Some audiologists, those with wonderful counseling skills, listen *through* the "information" question and answer it with an affective response, which is often just a simple "uh huh . . ."

Audiologists have the same emotions as all humans, of course, and usually have strong empathy for their patients. That empathy puts the audiologist's emotional wellness at risk. The audiologists who are best at counseling know this and are able to separate their behavior and affect toward the parent from their need to protect their own emotional wellness. They have extraordinary self-awareness of their nonverbal behaviors. They do not project defensiveness during these difficult conversations, and are not drawn in by the eagerness to answer a masked affective-question with an information-answer. Dr. David Luterman, professor of audiology at Emerson College in Boston and longtime guru in teaching counseling skills to audiologists, challenges the professional to listen to the parents in this time of crisis, and allow silence, or at most, a simple "uh huh" to be his or her response to these masked affective questions. In the space of quiet, the parent in crisis is allowed to fill the void with their denial, anger, bargaining, and any other normal reaction they may have to this abnormal situation.

Many well-meaning clinicians will tell parents going through this process "it's okay! He will be okay." Or will say something worse: "it's not as bad as it could be!" Or, they will overload the parents with information about how to manage this hearing loss. These are *not* examples of family-centered management. These are examples of the clinician responding to his or her own emotional needs by trying to lessen the pain the parent is experiencing and projecting to the empathic clinician. Alternatively, the clinician may respond in a very cold manner, showing no emotion and offering no witness or reflection of the parent's pain. A clinician has no right to attempt to lessen a parent's pain, or to protect himself or herself from the pain shared in empathy. It is the parent's right to feel the emotions he or she feels during and after these difficult conversations, and an attempt to ameliorate this pain, or put up an emotional wall, is to rob parents of their right to grieve and have the clinician bear witness to their grief. Everyone has a right to be heard, and to know that their feelings are important. It is the clinician's responsibility to hear the parent, and reinforce the importance of these awful feelings by bearing witness. It is a privilege to be allowed to share such an intimate, painful, life-changing event with a family, and the best audiologists know this. It took years of making mistakes, such as misinterpreting a masked affective question and giving it an information response, as well as careful mentoring by master clinicians, for me to begin to appreciate the privilege of sharing this moment with families.

Hopefully, parents of children with hearing loss reading this book experienced a supportive, emotionally available audiologist at the time of diagnosis. The conversation is never perfect, but hopefully it set the stage for family-centered intervention, given this was a medically driven diagnosis. Such is the new normal in pediatric audiology: parent-driven diagnosis and intervention is much less often encountered, thanks to universal newborn hearing screening. But the loss of the parent-driven path requires the family, not just the child, be the center of the intervention.

In our present society, a person need not have any hearing ability at all and live a happy, fulfilled life; extremely successful members of the Deaf community are testament to this. Historically, before rights to equal access for education and occupational opportunities were legislated, having childhood hearing loss presented insurmountable challenges. While it is easy to take for granted, the value of hearing cannot be easily overstated. Paraphrasing Helen Keller, "Deafness separates you from people; blindness separates you from things." With good hearing, spoken language develops effortlessly (all things being equal). Social and emotional attachments develop with deeper sincerity, as children become more sophisticated in their ability to express themselves. Affinity for music (from the Wiggles to Mozart to Justin Bieber) and dancing is apparent in babies from very early ages, and is a topic for friends to find common interest. From a basic safety perspective, threats (car horns on the highway or predators in the prehistoric forest) are heard from any direction, and before they can be seen.

Hearing loss that is present from birth (that is, the hearing loss is "congenital") is an invisible condition that (in the grand scheme) is not all that rare.[4] It risks creating enormous barriers between the baby's ability to reach her full educational, social, and emotional potential. If the hearing loss is identified quite early, and interventions start quickly, these barriers are often broken down quite successfully. If the hearing loss is not detected early, the barriers can disrupt the baby's ability to formulate his thoughts into meaningful chunks that is thought of as "symbolic language."[5] Lacking symbolic language, a toddler isn't able to request a bottle by expressing to his mother "baba!" (a protoword for "bottle"), or use the baby-sign for "milk": a hand-squeezing sign (which looks like milking a cow), requesting milk. Babies are born with brains that are primed to learn language, but language is not preprogrammed.

The language centers of the brain are awakened by stimulating them with meaningful exchanges of thought: usually, this is an automatic process with parents interacting with the baby during normal daily activities, like eating, bathing, reading, and playing. Parents automatically narrate what they are doing during these activities, and this verbal narration brings meaning to the areas of the baby's brain that develops and processes language. Babies' brains are also stimulated by eavesdropping on other family members' conversations. This "incidental learning" is the basis for babies starting to play with their own verbal sounds (that is, babbling), which is rewarded by parents who take delight in their baby's cute noises, raspberries, and squeals. With lots (and lots) of practice, these cute noises progress from nonsensical babbling ("babababa," "mamama") into more complex babbling ("mababamama") that starts to sound closer to a real word. Eventually, an actual linguistic "symbol" comes out, such as "baba," used to express a desire for a bottle (for instance). And that request is always "baba" and nothing else is "baba." Perhaps "mama" comes next (or "dada") and we have the makings of a very early vocabulary. It is an unbelievably proud day for parents of a toddler when these protowords are first uttered, marking a significant milestone in the child's development.

When hearing loss exists, the baby's ability to express himself or herself with meaningful chunks of thought is stymied. Depending on the severity of the hearing loss, the baby may not hear himself, and there is limited (or no) auditory feedback: the baby may not hear himself babble, and that detracts from the baby's joy of making sound. Babies with hearing loss do babble: it's fun to play with the vibration of the vocal cords and the lips and tongue. But there are subtle differences in the intonation of the babble of a baby with (untreated) hearing loss due to lack of auditory feedback on how his or her vocalizations sound.[6] Certainly, stimulation through sign language can assist in helping the baby with hearing loss (or with normal hearing) develop symbolic language: the squeezing hand motion for "milk" means the same thing whether the child can hear "Emma, do you want milk?" or not, if the sign is shown during the verbal utterance. If the child produces the sign for "milk" and is rewarded with milk, that behavior is reinforced and the child will consistently sign "milk" when that is her desired goal.

As the child grows older, for instance, age twelve months to twenty-four months, thoughts grow in complexity and the demands on language follow in kind. Children require of their caregivers a sounding board for their wants and needs. In a funny way, they are very self-centered and selfish at this stage. What if this complex thought is locked inside their heads without an avenue for expression? What a frustrating situation! Toddlers with undiagnosed/untreated hearing loss between twelve and twenty-four months often have marked behavioral challenges. Of course, toddlers with normal hearing who happen to be speech delayed also have behavioral challenges: just ask any parent whose toddler qualified for early intervention services and went from being a behavioral mess to reasonable with the institution of a few signs to reduce communication frustration.

EARLY LANGUAGE DEVELOPMENT, AND EARLY DIAGNOSIS OF PERMANENT HEARING LOSS

Imagine that before universal newborn hearing screening, it was between the ages of twelve and twenty-four months that parents became convinced that their child's communication challenges were a result of impaired hearing ability. What a validating feeling it must have been for parents to know that their suspicions were correct when the diagnosis was finally made! Over the past couple of decades, research by psychologist Patricia Kuhl, PhD, and audiologist Christine Yoshinaga-Itano, PhD, has informed us that, optimally, babies born with hearing loss should start receiving language intervention by six months of age. At six months, babies are just starting to sit up, unsupported, and are reliably sleeping through the night. They are nowhere near uttering their first word. It is ironic that the negative impact of childhood hearing loss is not typically experienced until long after this age, when the toddler fails to make good progress in spoken language development. But, all things being equal, by the time babies are six months old, they begin to develop an affinity for the speech sounds used in their native language. Psychologist Patricia Kuhl described babies younger than six months old as "citizens of the world." In her experiments in the 1970s and 1980s, the ability of a baby to detect a difference in the speech sound was determined using a pacifier with a special pressure sensor in it to tell when the baby was sucking, and when the baby's rhythm of sucking changed.[7] Babies would routinely suck on the pacifier, and would change the rhythm of their sucking when they noticed a change in sounds that were presented to them. For instance, Dr. Kuhl would play sounds like "dadadada" and measure the pacifier-sucking pattern of the infant. If the sound was changed from "dadada" to "mamama," the baby's pacifier-sucking pattern changed (suggesting the baby heard the difference). In babies under the age of six months, their sucking pattern changed easily with changes in speech sounds, no matter the language used. For instance, in babies raised in a family environment where a Western language (English) was spoken at home, the sucking rhythm changed when the sound "rarara" changed to "lalalala." The "ra" sound and "la" sound are not used in Eastern, tonal languages (like Cantonese, a Chinese dialect), but in babies raised in families speaking Cantonese, if they were *under* age six months, their pacifier-sucking behavior changed when the sound presented to them changed from "rarara" to "lalala." Conversely, in tonal languages, the "a" sound (as in "ma") changes the meaning quite significantly: one use of the word "ma" means mother, and a different inflection of the "a" in "ma" changes the meaning to "cow." Those raised using a Western language that does not make use of this change in vowel intonation simply do not "hear" the difference in the word, based on the change in the tone of the vowel. Young babies, under the age of six months, raised in Western-speaking homes, routinely changed their sucking rhythm when the sound "mamama" changed to a "mamama" (with different intonation on the "a"). However, when the experiment was repeated in babies six months and over, those raised in a Western language (e.g., English, which does not use different intonation of the "a" to indicate different meaning) no longer changed their pacifier-sucking pattern when the sound "mamama" changed to the different vowel "mamama." Those babies aged six months and over, raised in the Eastern language (e.g., Cantonese, which doesn't use "r" and "l") no longer switched up the rhythm of their pacifier-sucking when the sound "rarara" changed to "lalala." Dr. Kuhl concluded that babies under the age of six months were "citizens of the world" and were primed for being native language-learners if they were exposed to multiple languages from this very early age.

We can extrapolate this finding of "citizens of the world" to match with the findings of Dr. Christine Yoshinaga-Itano. In her ongoing studies of development of language in children with congenital hearing loss, she found that those infants identified with hearing loss before the age of six months developed language skills on par with their normal-hearing peers by the time they were three years old.[8] Those infants identified with hearing loss after six months continued to lag behind their normal hearing peers at age three years, suggesting that intervention for hearing loss should occur by age six months to provide children with hearing loss every opportunity to develop complex language matching their cognitive capabilities. In essence, the critical window for language development is open for the first six months of age, and, all things being equal with the child's cognitive ability, and other family factors, this window starts to close at age six months. Impressively, this window stays open for several years (we will discuss a possible age at which the window closes in a later chapter: but a brief spoiler—it could be as late as seven years old before the window actually closes on verbal language acquisition from auditory input).[9]

Since the advent of universal screening for hearing loss in newborns, it is now understood that congenital hearing loss is the most common sensory impairment, affecting three to four out of one thousand.[10] This is around sixteen thousand babies each year in the United States. The number of children with hearing loss increases throughout childhood and teenage years, with an estimated nineteen out of a thousand with hearing loss by age eighteen years.[11] Given the prevalence (that is, how common it is) for permanent childhood hearing loss, universal screening for hearing loss in newborns is standard of care in all states in the

United States, and most developed countries. Prior to the advent of universal newborn hearing screening, the average age of hearing loss diagnosis was two years old. With newborn hearing screening, some states are achieving an average age of diagnosis less than two months old. However, only six out of ten babies who do not pass the newborn hearing screening actually received diagnostic evaluations with an audiologist in a timely fashion. This is due in large part to challenges matching families with a qualified pediatric audiologist in a timely fashion, and the family being able to access that audiologist (who may be hundreds of miles away in large, Western states) for a condition that is not obvious in the newborn. This means that a large number of infants with hearing loss were initially flagged for further testing, but that further testing doesn't always happen. These children are then "late diagnosed" and remedial interventions are enacted, rather than proactive care that helps these children meet their developmental milestones.[12]

There is no magic age by which hearing loss diagnosis and intervention must happen. When possible, congenital hearing loss should be diagnosed as early as possible, and access to symbolic language (either sign, spoken, or both) be made accessible to the child. Family-centered intervention means the family, and the family's relationship with the baby, is at the core of all interventions to help the baby acquire language. This requires clinicians involved in the care of this child to understand the parent's experience, with regard to the diagnosis of hearing loss, and what that means to the parent's expectations of the child. Additionally, the dynamic within the extended family (grandparents, aunts and uncles, cousins) should be considered, because this is within the scope of this baby's influence. True family-centered intervention understands that the child with hearing loss does not develop a relationship with his world in the clinic, but in the day-to-day experiences with immediate and extended family. Ultimately, giving the child the avenue to explore her personality, and define her identity in this family unit (immediate and extended) is the goal of the clinicians involved in the care of the child with permanent, congenital hearing loss.

2

WHAT IS HEARING LOSS?
HOW DID THIS HAPPEN?

For the vast majority of us, we hear something twenty-four hours a day, seven days a week, from the moment we are born until the moment we die. Even if our hearing doesn't stay the same our whole lives (most of us do get some hearing loss, eventually), we often have at least some remaining hearing that registers what is happening around us. As simple and fundamental as hearing is to the majority of us, it is very easy to take for granted that it's actually a pretty complex process. The ear itself is a very impressive organ: we can hear across ten octaves of sound. For comparison, we can see across less than one octave of light. The range from the softest sound we can hear to the loudest we can tolerate and the dimmest light we can see to the brightest we can tolerate is similar. But our ears can handle huge changes in sound much more quickly than our eyes can adjust to even modest changes in brightness. It's a gift that we have the luxury to take this impressive sense for granted. When hearing loss happens, though, the value of the gift becomes much more obvious.

In this chapter, we consider what it might be like to have hearing loss, how hearing loss is defined, and what are the causes in children. Some of the material in this chapter gets a bit technical, particularly when I talk about the parts of the ear that can be affected, and the kind of hearing loss that results. If any of the material creates more questions than answers, I encourage you to bring these questions to someone knowledgeable about the medical aspects of hearing. Most healthcare providers welcome the opportunity to teach, especially when there are specific questions that can help improve communication between the family and providers. Bridging the knowledge gaps between members of the team taking care of a child with hearing loss helps to focus interventions on being family-centered.

WHAT IS IT LIKE TO HAVE HEARING LOSS?

It can be hard to thoroughly understand what it's like to have hearing loss, unless you have hearing loss yourself. Plugging your ears with your fingers barely gives a "mild" hearing loss, and having no hearing (e.g., "profound" hearing loss) is the far opposite end of that range; there is a very large range of hearing sensitivity in between. Even for people who have hearing loss, each person experiences his or her hearing loss uniquely: this is because the ear is a doorway for meaningful sound to reach the brain. We actually hear with our brains, more than we do with our ears.

Differences from unique experiences acknowledged, there are similar challenges for people with similar degrees of hearing loss. Contrary to common knowledge, the degree of hearing loss isn't described as a percent of loss; there's no "50 percent hearing loss." Instead, hearing loss is defined by categories according to the expected difficulty hearing and understanding speech. In order of increasing degree of difficulty, hearing-loss severity is described as: mild, moderate, severe, and profound. Hearing loss often affects different pitches to different degrees. That is, hearing loss might be more mild in lower pitches (think of the keys on a piano on the left side of the keyboard) and more severe in the higher pitches (such as the piano keys on the right side of the keyboard). Hearing loss might be less severe in one ear and more severe in the other. Also, just because a sound is loud enough for the person with hearing loss to hear, that does not mean the brain is able to make sense of the sound.[1]

Hearing loss interferes with the ear's ability to provide the brain with access to the meaningful sounds of speech. How much interference depends how much hearing loss, and what pitches are affected. When hearing loss affects the higher pitches more than the lower pitches, as it often does, vowel sounds (a, e, i, o, u) are more audible than consonant sounds (for instance, f, th, p, k, h). The result might be like the teacher's voice in Charlie Brown cartoons ("Wah, wah-wah, wah-wah"): the person with this hearing loss can tell a person is talking, but not be able to understand what was said.

Let's take a visual comparison of hearing loss. In figure 2.1 below is a sentence, repeated, starting with "profound" loss of access to the words, followed by "severe," then "moderate" then "mild." For sake of sharing this experience with me and all readers, pull out a bookmark or index card, and cover all the examples, and slide it down to reveal only one more example at a time, starting from the top.

With a profound loss, there is essentially a blank space. The period is left at the end to offer a little guidance where that sentence ends. In the severe loss example, the letters of the words are so faint that you might not be able to make out that there are words. Unless your lighting is extremely good and your eyesight is excellent, you probably cannot read the words, or even tell there are words there. In the moderate loss, some of the letters are dark enough against the white page for you to make out there are words, and some idea where words start and the next begins. But likely you can't read the sentence and understand it. In the mild loss visual example, if your eyesight and the lighting is adequate, you can make out most of the letters, but not all. Perhaps you can piece together the meaning of the sentence, filling in the gaps where some of the consonant sounds are still too faint to make out. If this sentence were part of a paragraph, and you followed the gist of that paragraph (even though the whole paragraph would have words with blanks in them), you could probably understand everything. Finally, the normal example clarifies all the letters. At what "severity" of loss of visual input were you able to correctly identify all the letters in each word?

The example above has no background "noise" to interfere with the contrast between the letters and the blank page. This is like having a hearing loss, and listening to the sentence spoken in a quiet room. If there is some background interference, it can make the letters more challenging to decipher.

In this next example, I'll add some visual "noise" to another sentence, repeated, from profound loss to normal (figure 2.2). The "noise" in this example includes both background random noise (like the noise from an air conditioner or noisy radiator) and random sentences unrelated to our target sentence in our example. The random noise and visual "babble" are both distracting, and make it harder to make out the words of our target sentence. You'll also notice the severity of the loss affects both the target sentence and the noise, but even so, the loss of contrast between the target sentence and the background noise make it much harder to make out "moderate" and "mild" than in the first example above (with no background noise). Use your bookmark or index card

Profound loss:
┌───┐
│   .   │
└───┘

Severe loss:
┌───┐
│ I ave wri en   e ire ion on   e a   of i   ar .   │
└───┘

Moderate loss:
┌───┐
│ I ave wri en the dire ions on the ba   of this ard.   │
└───┘

Mild loss:
┌───┐
│ I have written the directions on the back of this card.   │
└───┘

Normal:
┌───┐
│ I have written the directions on the back of this card.   │
└───┘

Figure 2.1.   Visual analogy of hearing loss, with no background "noise"

again to reveal only one more example at a time, starting from profound loss.

If your vision and reading abilities are normal, you should have been able to read the "mild" loss example with no background noise, and perhaps the moderate loss example. In the background noise example, it was probably too hard to read anything but the normal example. However, you probably could read the normal example with only a little difficulty.

When a person has hearing loss, no one else around them automatically knows. Since most people (especially children and young adults) have normal hearing, we all expect people we talk with to have hearing in the "normal" range. Even in significant background noise, people with normal hearing can follow along (just like in our "normal" visual example with background noise). Consider the disconnect that would likely happen if your expectations were that the person you are talking

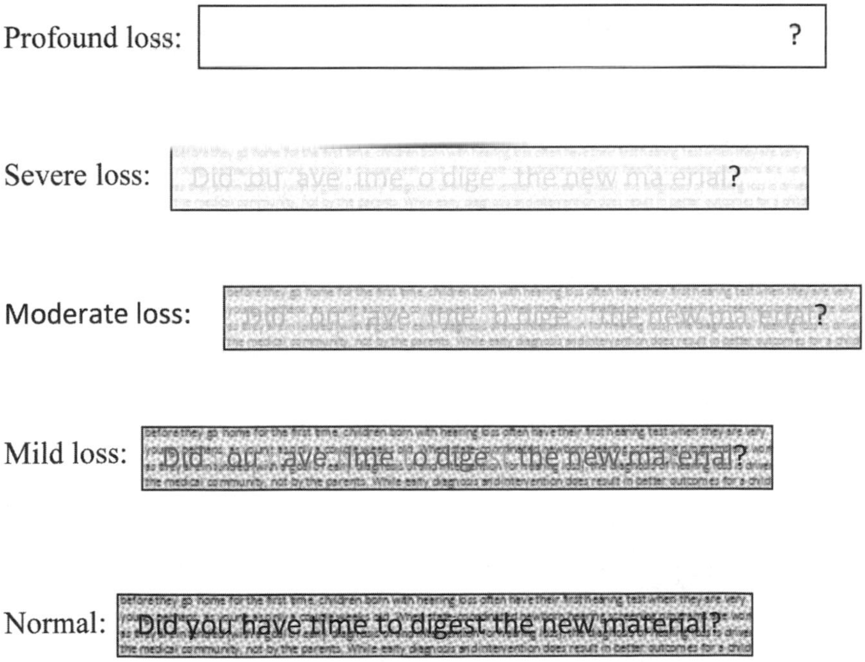

Profound loss:

Severe loss:

Moderate loss:

Mild loss:

Normal:

Figure 2.2. Visual analogy of hearing loss, *with* added background "noise"

with had normal hearing, but instead they had a moderate hearing loss. She would catch some of what you said, but certainly not all. If it's quiet, and she asks you to repeat yourself and she focuses and thinks really hard, she will probably be able to figure out what you said. And that would be exhausting, over time. Since it's so exhausting to try to keep up, most people with this degree of (untreated) hearing loss try to fill in the gaps (and often guess wrong) or try to dictate the conversation. People having the conversation with them will most likely mistake the inappropriateness for something other than hearing loss: he isn't paying attention to me; he isn't very bright; he is very bossy and boisterous. It is a sad irony that the attempts the person with hearing loss will make to stay engaged can drive others away.

If the person had a mild hearing loss, and it was quiet, likely she could keep up with the conversation more easily, and it would be less taxing than for the person with moderate hearing loss. If the person had a severe or profound hearing loss, she might follow if she is especially good at speech-reading (i.e., lip reading) and using visual cues to catch the meaning; but it is unlikely hearing is adding anything to her ability to follow what is spoken. If it's noisy, even the person with mild hearing loss would probably be incapable of following, and asking for you to repeat yourself would yield the same challenging attempt to understand . . . which would quickly become too frustrating to keep trying to talk, for both of you.

If the person with hearing loss doesn't get help to hear better, this disconnect and frustration would naturally be very isolating. In speaking with young, successful adults with hearing loss, the scariest part of their experience with hearing loss is the isolation they feel when they can't keep up with a conversation, when everyone else (with normal hearing) takes for granted how easy it is for them to decode the conversation. When a large group of people socialize together (think of a Super Bowl party at home or at a bar), it's typically quite noisy and there is rapid change of topics from one conversation to another, with multiple, unrelated conversations happening at the same time. The same is true at many holiday parties and family get-togethers. A person with hearing loss, who finds it difficult to follow a single conversation with only a little background noise, would find these big social events incompatible with his listening ability (but not his ability to add to the conversation, if only he had the means to do so). And so, even though he is surrounded by people, he is, in essence, by himself. Isolated.

It's no wonder, then, that people with hearing loss prefer smaller social groups and often have a small circle of close friends. Many people (normal hearing or not) prefer a few very close friends; other people who have a natural gregariousness to them might want to be the "life of the party" and socialize with as many people as possible. For young people with hearing loss who have a natural "life of the party" spark in them, their hearing loss might force them into socializing in a way that doesn't match with a naturally outgoing nature. It is also no wonder that many people with hearing loss get married to someone who also has hearing loss, particularly those who identify culturally with the Deaf community (using American Sign Language and typically do not use hearing as part of navigating their lives). The circle of friends and acquaintances may well be considerably smaller for the person with hearing loss than for a peer with normal hearing; but within the smaller circle, each member finds solace from the isolation.

So far in this chapter, the impact of hearing loss has been described using visual examples for a person who has long been a fluent communicator (you, the reader, are fluent enough in written English to read this book). With a lifetime of using English behind you, you can fill in many gaps in understanding. We all do this routinely, every day, without even realizing it. Let's turn attention then to a child with hearing loss; specifically, a child who has not yet learned language. Maybe a reasonable analogy would be for an adult who is fluent only in English trying to learn to read Italian with all the consonants faded, relative to the vowels. It would be insurmountably challenging for most of us.

In a child with just about any degree of hearing loss, learning to decode the pops, squeaks, and hums that make up the sounds of spoken language is equally insurmountably challenging if the hearing loss goes undetected or the hearing loss is detected, but appropriate intervention isn't accessed. The brain is primed for language, but the door bringing the meaningful sound to the brain is too closed for language to be acquired naturally. And just like in the example above, the expectation is that hearing is normal, and so a disconnect happens between the expected outcome (learning to talk) and reality (speech delay). This disconnect results in the child being unable to express increasingly complex thoughts as her brain matures and her wants, needs, and personality become more mature as she grows from an infant into a toddler. The inability of children with hearing loss to express themselves very often means behavioral challenges (think inconsolable and unreasonable toddler freaking out, often) and interference with family relationships.

DIFFERENT TYPES OF HEARING LOSS

Similar to there being different degrees of hearing loss severity, there are different types of hearing loss. To understand the different types of hearing loss, first we need to understand the basic parts of the ear. Figure 2.3 is a picture of the ear, which has three major sections: the outer ear, the middle ear, and the inner ear. The outer ear is made of the pinna ("PINN-uh"; the part of the ear on the side of our head) and the ear canal, ending with the eardrum. The middle ear is made of an air-filled pocket on the other side of the eardrum and the three smallest bones in our body (the ossicles: the malleus, the incus, and the stapes) and ends with the base (the "footplate") of the stapes, last and smallest of the three ossicles. The inner ear is made of the cochlea, the vestibule, and the semicircular canals. The cochlea is quite small: it's roughly the size of a green pea, and is coiled up like a snail shell. The cochlea is where the sound that comes in from the outer ear and goes through the middle ear gets turned into nerve signals, which are sent to the brain by the auditory nerve; in essence, the cochlea "hears" and the brain "listens." The outer and middle ear is a pathway for the sound in our environment to get to our cochlea. The other parts of the inner ear (the vestibule and semicircular canals) participate in our balance system, specifically by telling the balance centers in the brain the position of our head (Are you looking up or down?) and if we are moving (Are you spinning around, or moving straight ahead?). In children, the balance system is very important for learning to walk (as well as hitting many other gross motor milestones).

There are two main types of hearing loss: *conductive* ("con-DUCK-tiv") and *sensorineural* ("SENSE-ory-NOO-ral"). A conductive hearing loss blocks sound going through the outer and middle ear from getting to the cochlea at the same loudness level (that is, intensity). A conductive hearing loss can be caused by something as simple as a plug of earwax completely blocking the ear canal. This acts like an earplug, and could drop hearing from normal into the mild hearing-loss range. As expected, this kind of hearing loss is temporary, and is easily treated by removing the earwax. Another very common cause of conductive hearing loss in children is the fluid that builds up inside the middle ear when there is an ear infection. This fluid might be thin and watery (think of a runny nose, with clear nasal discharge) or could be thick

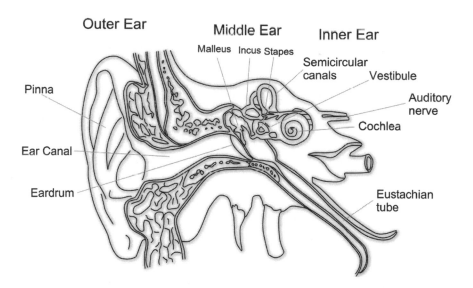

Figure 2.3.   Parts of the ear (copyright Boscorelli) Copyright Boscorelli/ 123RF.com

mucous (think of nasal discharge from a sinus infection). The hearing loss resulting from fluid is often mild, but could be in the moderate hearing-loss range. It is temporary, acting like an earplug (or "hearing underwater") while the fluid is there. Once the infection clears up, the fluid should clear up too, and hearing improves. In 10 percent of children under the age of four years, they get enough ear infections that their hearing fluctuates from normal to mild hearing loss often enough that it interferes with them consistently hearing all the speech sounds, and can cause a speech delay.[2] Ear infections are most common in children aged eighteen months to two-and-a-half years, and become much less common in children aged seven years and up. Not all ear infections result in the classic symptoms of fever, ear pain, loss of appetite, irritability, and obvious hearing loss. Sometimes, the body's immune system (and/or antibiotics used to treat the infection) succeed in killing the bacteria causing the infection, but the fluid lingers. Fluid might be present without there being pain or fever, and so the fluid can cause a (temporary) hearing loss that goes undetected. The American Academy of Pediatrics has issued recommendations for when a child with ear infections should be referred to an ear, nose, and throat physician (an "otolaryngologist") for consideration of more aggressive medical treatment of ear infections (http://pediatrics.aappublications.org/content/early/2013/02/20/peds.2012-3488).[3]

These common examples of temporary causes of conductive hearing loss (earwax impaction and fluid from ear infections) can interfere significantly with a child's hearing ability. Conductive hearing loss makes all sound quieter: louder sounds are made softer, and quieter sounds are made even quieter (and easily too soft to be heard). This is particularly problematic in children in early elementary school, when ear infections are still relatively common and children are learning the fundamentals of reading and writing. Lingering middle-ear fluid causes a mild hearing loss, and this mild hearing loss causes the distance over which the child can hear to get much smaller than when the child's hearing is normal. For instance, a child with normal hearing can adequately hear a teacher from twelve feet away, as long as the classroom is quiet. A child with a mild conductive hearing loss might need to be no further than three feet away from the teacher in order to adequately hear the teacher.

Most of the time, children are not born with a conductive hearing loss. In the relatively rare event a child is born with conductive hearing loss (that is, their hearing loss is "congenital"—that is, "present at birth"), it is because of a structural issue with the outer or middle ear, or both. The ear canal might not have fully formed during pregnancy, or may not have formed at all. This is called "ear canal atresia" or an "atretic ear canal." Sometimes, children with ear canal atresia also have incompletely formed pinna. When the pinna is not completely formed, this is called "microtia." Most of the time, one ear is affected and the other ear is unaffected. Sometimes, both ears are affected, but one ear is more obviously affected than the other. If the outer ear is incompletely formed, it is common for the bones of the middle ear to also be incompletely formed. During my career as a pediatric audiologist, I have seen two children (we'll call them Karen and Arthur) who were born with microtia and atresia on one side (that is "unilateral"), but had "bilateral" (that is, both ears) hearing loss. The side with the incompletely formed pinna and ear canal had the attention of all the care providers, and as one would expect, the obviously incompletely formed side had significant hearing loss (in both cases, the degree of hearing loss in the obviously affected ear was moderate-to-severe conductive hearing loss). However, in the other ear, with the normal-looking pinna and ear canal, there was incomplete formation of the ossicles, and a mild-to-moderate conductive hearing loss existed. In one child, Karen, the hearing loss in the "better" ear was not discovered until she was sixteen months old, when she came to see me as part of her overall evaluations to help her care team advise the family what could be done for her "poorer" ear. She had not had a newborn hearing screening, since it was obvious she would not pass the screening in the ear with microtia and atresia. Unfortunately, her medical team assumed that meant hearing in her nonatretic (well-appearing ear) was normal, and so the hearing screening (and follow-up hearing testing) were deferred

while attention was given to figuring out if any other organs had problems. In the second child, Arthur, his bilateral hearing loss was diagnosed in his first few weeks of life, as he saw me for hearing evaluation
after not passing newborn hearing screening in either ear. While we
aren't covering hearing loss treatment in this chapter, I'll divulge: both
children were fitted with a hearing aid in their more completely formed
ear within weeks after diagnosis of hearing loss in both ears. Karen's
spoken language came along very quickly after being fitted with amplification, since her cochlea on that side had always been good, and she
had been able to hear her own vocal sounds inside her head all along.
Now she heard outside her head much better, and her brain made good
sense of those sounds and this supported her acquisition of spoken
language. Arthur was still quite young when he started using the hearing aid in his more completely formed ear, and he had several other
medical challenges. While these other medical challenges took first priority (over his speech development), he has made good progress with
spoken language as of the time of this book's writing.

When there is a congenital "permanent" conductive hearing loss
(that is, conductive hearing loss due to incomplete formation of the
outer and/or middle ear), the cause is often unknown. Sometimes it
happens without any other organs or systems in the body being affected, and sometimes the incomplete ear formation happens along
with other systems forming incorrectly. When other systems are involved, the child may be diagnosed with a "syndrome" (which is simply
the medical term for a condition where two or more of the body's
systems are not working correctly and they share the same root cause).
A syndrome might be a chance happening, and not a trait inherited
from either parent. Other times, the syndrome might be inherited
through the genes from one or both parents. If the syndrome is due to
genes the child inherited, there is a chance of them passing those genes
to any of their children. Regardless of the cause of the permanent
conductive hearing loss, just how permanent the loss is depends in part
on whether or not the structural issues can be addressed at some point

by surgery to improve the function of the affected part of the ear. We will discuss this more extensively in chapter 6.

Hearing loss stemming from an issue with how well the cochlea works is termed sensorineural hearing loss. A somewhat antiquated, but still occasionally used, term for sensorineural hearing loss is "nerve deafness." Later in this chapter, we'll discuss hearing loss due to problems specifically with the auditory nerve; the hearing loss resulting from an issue with the auditory nerve is distinctly different from the hearing loss resulting from issues with the cochlea. Cochlear hearing loss is also distinctly different from conductive hearing loss. A plug of earwax, or hearing underwater due to middle-ear fluid, affects soft through loud sounds pretty much the same: it makes all sound quieter by the same amount (that is, by the amount of hearing loss: typically, a mild decrease in audibility). When a person has sensorineural hearing loss stemming from a problem with the cochlea, sounds that are above the threshold of hearing (that is, sound that is louder than the softest sound he or she can hear) are *just as loud* to the person with hearing loss as a person with normal hearing. Sounds that are near the threshold of hearing are much softer to the person with hearing loss than the person with normal hearing. Sounds that are below the threshold of hearing simply aren't there for the person with hearing loss. A visual example of a conductive hearing loss would be like all letters in the words being printed dimmer by the same amount. In a sensorineural hearing loss, some letters are just as dark as in the "normal" sentence example while others are very dim and some are absent.

Actual audio examples of conductive and sensorineural hearing loss are available through simulation software. These simulations are of var-

Mild to moderate sensorineural hearing loss: | The gol er ried o ma e is u . |

Normal: | The golfer tried to make his putt. |

Figure 2.4.   Visual analogy of mild to moderate sensorineural hearing loss

ying accuracy, so it is best to seek guidance from reputable sources. I have several examples of conductive and sensorineural hearing loss on my practice's website (www.bosaudconsult.com).

WHO HAS PERMANENT HEARING LOSS, AND WHY?

Sensorineural hearing loss is most often permanent, rather than temporary. In adults, the number-one cause of hearing loss is aging, followed by chronic exposure to high-level noise. Hearing loss is the third most common chronic health condition in people over the age of sixty-five years, more common than diabetes and heart disease. In newborns, permanent sensorineural hearing loss is present in about three of every one thousand babies in developed countries, like the United States (it's more common than this in the developing world).[4] Three out of a thousand may not sound like a very big number, but is the most common congenital sensory challenge (markedly more common than low vision) and far more common than many other significant health conditions present at birth, such as cleft lip or palate, Down syndrome, and metabolic disorders. For frame of reference, roughly six babies per one thousand are born extremely premature (less than twenty-eight weeks gestational age).[5] Half of all babies born with hearing loss have no indications for hearing loss, or any other medical issues. This half of babies born with hearing loss are born full-term, healthy, and have the usual thirty-six- to forty-eight-hour stay in the hospital before going home with parents. Ninety percent of children born with hearing loss have parents with normal hearing, and there is no history of childhood permanent hearing loss. It is especially important for this group of healthy children that newborn hearing screening be completed prior to the baby leaving the hospital, since this is the group of children most at risk for hearing loss going undetected until the child is a toddler. These children also have no other medical or developmental issues that would hold them back from achieving their full social, emotional, and educational potential, and so perhaps they stand to benefit the most from early detection of hearing loss.

For the other half of babies born with hearing loss and medical problems, many of them are born prematurely, have breathing problems, have low birth weight, and may have infections that must be treated aggressively. Most often, these babies will be treated in a neonatal intensive care unit (NICU), which is a specialized care facility for newborns within hospitals. Once these babies recover and are discharged home, they are referred to as "NICU graduates." Hearing screening and hearing-loss intervention understandably takes a back seat to more pressing, life-threatening medical problems when the baby is in the NICU. However, hearing loss is much more common in NICU graduates than in babies without medical problems; it is estimated that one to two out of one hundred NICU graduates have hearing loss (nearly ten times as common as the three per one thousand in the well-baby group).[6] Once the baby being cared for in the NICU is "out of the woods" and medical care turns from "rescue" and into "recovery," these children also tend to make exceptional developmental strides despite their hearing loss, with appropriate intervention. NICU graduates with hearing loss tend to differ from those babies with hearing loss born full-term and healthy, as the children who had a challenging start to life are often already well connected with the medical community. Addressing the diagnosis and intervention for hearing loss either becomes part of the "whole package" or takes a back seat to the other, ongoing medical concerns.

The most common cause of permanent, sensorineural hearing loss in healthy newborns is genetic inheritance from both parents.[7] Specifically, there are genes (the "Connexin" genes) that are responsible for making the cochlea manage the correct concentration of potassium (a nutrient the cochlea needs to work correctly). If one parent carries a gene that cannot correctly code for the system that is needed to manage nutrient concentration in the cochlea, but the other parent does, then the child will have cochleas that do their job. If both parents carry this aberrant gene and it is passed along to the child, then the child's genes encode a system that cannot correctly manage potassium concentrations. The end result is a child whose cochleas don't work very well, but the child is expected to be otherwise very healthy.

Another fairly common cause of congenital, sensorineural hearing loss is a viral infection picked up while the mother was pregnant. It is estimated that 1 percent of all babies are born after their mother contracted cytomegalovirus ("SEYE-toe-MEGALO-virus"; abbreviated CMV) for the first time while pregnant. CMV is very common, with around 40 percent of adults carrying the virus.[8] Typically, when first contracting the virus, it makes us a little under the weather, like we have a cold. Once you catch it and your body fights off the infection, you carry the virus for the rest of your life, but it can't affect you anymore. CMV infection is only truly concerning when a mother who is pregnant never had CMV before, and contracts the virus during pregnancy. CMV infection during pregnancy can cause the loss of the pregnancy, or cause the baby to be born prematurely. Sometimes (5 to 10 percent of the time) the baby with congenital CMV is born ill and requires NICU care. Most often, the baby is born otherwise healthy, but may have developmental challenges that become apparent during childhood: sensorineural hearing loss, cognitive impairment, vision impairment, and seizure disorder, for instance. In fact, sensorineural hearing loss is the most common problem that can arise from congenital CMV.

An unfortunate aspect of congenital CMV infection is that if the child develops sensorineural hearing loss, it is not always present immediately at birth. In fact, in children who end up having sensorineural hearing loss due to congenital CMV infection, half of them have normal hearing at birth, with the hearing loss setting in months or years later. These "delayed-onset" hearing losses would be missed by newborn hearing screening, but still likely interfere with the child learning to talk. In fact, passing the newborn hearing screening can give the family and care providers a false sense of security! During my postdoctoral fellowship at Boston Children's Hospital, my colleagues and I studied causes of delayed-onset hearing loss and timing of diagnosis; when a child had a hearing screening and passed, but had a delayed-onset hearing loss, the child wouldn't be diagnosed and treated as early as those children who never had a hearing screening before going home from the hospital. Our interpretation was that passing a newborn hearing screening resulted in delayed diagnosis and intervention in children who have delayed-onset hearing loss. Just because a child passes the newborn hearing screening does not mean he or she is "vaccinated" against a future hearing loss.

The American Academy of Pediatrics has a wealth of information about congenital CMV infection. A fact sheet about congenital CMV (prepared by a guru in congenital CMV infection, Dr. Susan Fowler of the University of Alabama) can be found at http://www.aap.org/en-us/advocacy-and-policy/aap-health-initiatives/PEHDIC/Documents/CMV.pdf.

There are many other reasons why a child's hearing may change. While it is rare for a child to be born with normal hearing and then hearing decrease early in life, it can happen. It is fairly common for the hearing of a child born with hearing loss to progressively decrease. In addition to congenital CMV infection, other reasons hearing loss progresses includes significant breathing problems at birth (problems bad enough to require mechanical ventilation for more than five days), serious infections requiring aggressive use of a certain class of antibiotics (the "aminoglycoside" family of antibiotics), and subtle errors in the formation of the temporal bone where the cochlea and vestibular system organs reside in the skull.[9] The temporal bone is the part of the skull on the side of the head; it has cavities and channels running through it (some of which make up structures of the ear). If certain errors happen when parts of the baby's ear and skull are forming in the womb, it can result in an ear with hearing loss, or with an ear with normal hearing but a predisposition to delayed onset and progressive hearing loss. These errors are collective termed "temporal bone malformations" and the ones that specifically affect hearing are Enlarged Vestibular Aqueduct (EVA) and Mondini malformation. These malformations are very subtle, and can't be seen by looking at the baby or physically examining the head. They can only be identified on a high-resolution CT scan (a very powerful type of X-ray) or MRI of the side of the head.

It is also possible that the baby's ear can be injured, resulting in hearing loss. Hearing loss caused by high level sound, termed "noise-induced hearing loss" ("NIHL") is very common in adults, but uncommon in babies. However, it can happen, and it is not clear if the baby's ear is more susceptible to being damaged by high-level sound than an adult's. Quick rule of thumb: if it's too loud to carry a conversation, it's too loud for a baby to be in that noisy area.[10] Other injuries that are perhaps more obvious are from a head injury, particularly resulting in a skull fracture. Automobile accidents, falls from a height taller than the child, and unsecured furniture (bookshelves or televisions) toppling over when a toddler tries to climb up are common causes of skull fractures that can lead to permanent hearing loss. Last, while uncommon for an infant or very young child to need cancer treatments, the backbone chemotherapy drugs used to fight cancerous tumors, cisplatinum ("SIS-PLAT-in-um") and carboplatinum ("CARBO-plat-in-um"), are toxic to the cochlea. It is extremely common for a child being treated for cancer to require frequent hearing tests to monitor hearing during chemotherapy treatment, in order to guide the oncologists (cancer specialists) in understanding the side effects of the cancer treatments. It is the oncologists' dilemma, to have to rely on certain drugs to save a child's life, but risk causing a permanent condition that can interfere with speech-language acquisition and impact quality of life.[11]

With advancements in hearing-test equipment that allows us to tease out how different parts of the ear function independently from the other parts, a hearing disorder called Auditory Neuropathy Spectrum Disorder (ANSD) has been identified.[12] This hearing disorder has actually always been around, but our ability to test for it came about in the 1990s. This disorder is also referred to as Auditory Neuropathy (AN) and Auditory Dys-synchrony (AD). Historically, hearing tests could determine how much conductive and how much sensorineural hearing loss was present. The sensorineural component of the hearing loss reflected everything from the cochlea up to the brain. With newer technology (namely, otoacoustic emissions and Auditory Brainstem Response, which we will cover in detail in chapter 3), audiologists can tease out what happens in the cochlea (the "sensory" part of sensorineural) and what happens above the cochlea (the "neural" part of sensorineural). In classic cases of ANSD, the middle ear and cochlea are working just fine, but the connection between the cochlea and the hearing nerve has a problem with it. The hearing nerve is supposed to fire in an organized fashion when the sound reaching the cochlea is loud enough. When ANSD happens, the nerve doesn't fire in an organized fashion, and instead of a clear signal going from the ear to the brain, a very distorted and fuzzy signal travels up the nerves. The result is that sounds to a person with ANSD may be loud enough for them to hear, but the signal going up to the brain is too muddled for them to make use of it. This specific hearing disorder (actual "nerve" deafness) creates fairly significant challenges for intervention, because it is (most often) permanent, and the tests used to figure out the degree of hearing loss are not able to describe how severe the ANSD is impacting speech understanding. When working with a family to manage the impact of hearing loss due to ANSD, the audiologists don't have all the usual tools to guide his or her recommendations. This hearing disorder is the least common of the types of hearing disorders: it is estimated that one in ten children with profound hearing loss actually have ANSD, rather than a cochlear hearing loss. The causes are less well known than for cochlear hearing loss, but babies born at less than twenty-eight weeks gestational age ("extreme prematurity") and those with high jaundice (significantly elevated bilirubin levels) are thought to be at greater risk for ANSD. While ANSD creates some complications to the audiologist figuring out how best to improve meaningful access to language, thankfully the hearing healthcare professions have enough experience now to make confident recommendations for fitting of devices to maximize hearing, and to support children's acquisition of language, regardless of what type of hearing loss they have.

The list of reasons for the cause of permanent childhood hearing loss is long, and many of the causes are dangerous to the whole child, not just his or her hearing. For the most part, when a sensorineural hearing loss is diagnosed, it is not amenable to medical or surgical interventions, and so is considered "permanent." However, the hearing loss itself does not "hurt." It is not physically painful. The hearing loss creates a potential barrier to communication, and it is typically an invisible barrier. The good news is that clinical science has found exceptionally good techniques for screening for hearing loss at any age, diagnosing the hearing loss at any age, and providing timely intervention to break down the potential communication barriers.

3

HOW HEARING IS TESTED IN INFANTS AND YOUNG CHILDREN

In this chapter, we detail the goals of early detection of hearing loss and what constitutes "early." There are several different ways hearing can be tested, and the abbreviations for all these different tests are like alphabet soup. In this chapter, we focus on how the different kinds of hearing tests are conducted, and why they are important. Finally, we go through what the test results mean and how they are used to direct next steps.

It is now standard of care for babies to have their hearing screened by the age of one month, those with hearing loss diagnosed with the condition by three months of age, and intervention to break down the communication barriers by six months of age. In addition, monitoring children for signs of hearing loss and timely identification and intervention of delayed-onset hearing loss is another core principle of the currently accepted standard of care. These principles of "1-3-6" (the age, in months, by which a child has been screened, diagnosed, and received intervention for hearing loss) have been driven by the most recent position statement (2007) of the Joint Committee on Infant Hearing (JCIH).[1] The JCIH is an active working group, made of representatives from several professional organizations (including pediatrics, ENT, audiology, speech-language pathology, and deaf education) as well as representatives from the Deaf community, state and federal health and welfare agencies (including the US Centers for Disease Control and Prevention), and supporting academic institutions. They are charged with providing interdisciplinary leadership in establishing policy that guides standard of care for diagnosis and intervention for childhood hearing loss, based on periodic review of advancements in research and technology. Long story short: when someone says "they say this is how things should be done for babies with hearing loss," the JCIH is the "*they*"—the group of experts who set the bar for how to do things the right way.

The JCIH was first formed in 1969 based in large part on the tireless efforts of Dr. Marion Downs, *the* pioneering pediatric audiologist.[2] Dr. Downs developed techniques for screening newborns via noise makers and observing their behavioral responses in the early 1960s. It is now understood that even newborns with normal hearing do not reliably show how good their hearing is; that said, Dr. Downs's efforts were the first time anyone had tried to identify hearing loss in babies this young. Concurrently, she promoted the fitting of hearing aids to babies with hearing loss as young as six months of age, at a time when most children with hearing loss were not diagnosed with hearing loss and fitted with hearing aids until they were two to three years old. At the time, skeptics considered intervening earlier than this a fool's errand. Over time, research has validated Dr. Downs's groundbreaking theories, that early diagnosis and intervention is possible and this results in markedly better outcomes than waiting until the child is a toddler. Dr. Downs received numerous awards and recognition, including the Marion Downs Hearing Center at the University of Colorado Medical Center named in her honor, as well as two honorary doctoral degrees. She passed away on November 13, 2014, at the age of one hundred; she will be remembered as the driving force behind universal screening of newborns for hearing loss to provide timely and appropriate intervention (www.mariondowns.com).

Newborns do alert to sound, and can even turn their heads to the side where a sound is presented. They quiet to their mother's voice, which is not surprising, since they have been listening to their mother's

voice from inside the womb since they were only twenty weeks gestational age.[3] But they don't do this consistently. At least, not consistently
enough to use a newborn's behavior to tell what he or she can and
cannot hear. But our ears, nerves, and brain give off tiny signals when
hearing "happens," and these can be observed and recorded using very
sensitive test equipment. This observation and recording is an "objective" test of the function of hearing. In the early 1990s, it became
technically feasible to perform this test of nerve signals associated with
hearing on a broad scale (that is, for all newborns). In 1994, the JCIII
published a position statement calling for the universal screening of
newborns via objective test measures.[4] What is considered "standard of
care" by JCIH has been updated twice since, to clarify how and when
screening (and diagnosis and intervention) should happen. In 2014,
newborn hearing screening is a mature public health initiative, achieving relatively universal provision throughout the United States and
many developed countries. In many states in the United States, more
than 95 percent of newborns are screened for hearing loss before they
go home from the birth hospital. Early diagnosis and intervention isn't
there yet, though. Areas still in need of improvement are the diagnosis
of hearing loss by age three months, and intervention by age six
months.[5]

A screening is just that, though: a *screening*. It is a quick test designed to raise suspicion that further, more detailed testing is needed to
uncover true hearing abilities. Either they "pass" the screening (and
don't need further testing), or they "refer" for further testing. Often,
screening tests are reported as "pass" or "fail." However, "fail" is an
incorrect way to say it (you don't "fail and refer for testing," you simply
"refer for testing"). Additionally, the word "fail" carries with it such a
negative emotional burden for new parents. "Your baby failed" is neither technically correct, nor a positive and motivating thing to say to
parents. The vast majority of parents of children with hearing loss I
have spoken with about this topic have said they had a bad experience
with being told their baby didn't pass the hearing screening. Often, the
results were communicated in a way that downplayed the importance:

"Don't worry, it's probably just fluid." Other times, the parents are told in a way that totally freaked the parents out, prematurely (and unnecessarily): "Well, since he failed he might need a hearing aid." Both extremes are remembered with bitterness by parents of children who went on to be diagnosed with hearing loss. A better way parents could be told their baby didn't pass the screening might be like this: "Your baby didn't pass the hearing screening, so we don't know how good the baby's hearing is yet. We've scheduled an appointment with an audiologist in three weeks, where they'll do the testing needed to find out just how good his hearing is."

A screening is not meant to give all the answers right away; further specialized testing is necessary to determine how good hearing is when a newborn doesn't pass the hearing screening in one or both ears. In reality, roughly one in twelve newborns who don't pass a hearing screen in one ear but pass in the other end up having hearing loss (sometimes hearing loss in both ears, despite that they screen in only one ear). One in three newborns who don't pass the hearing screening in both ears end up having hearing loss (very often, in both). In total, between the one-ear refers and bilateral refers, roughly one of every five who don't pass the screening have hearing loss. So, four out of five have normal hearing, but the screening doesn't show how good the hearing really was. Chances are, if a baby doesn't pass the hearing screening (in either or both ears), the baby turns out to have normal hearing. But the odds are not so favorable that follow-up testing can be skipped, or can wait until the baby is much older.

While more than 95 percent of newborns are screened in most states in the United States, less than 60 percent of those who don't pass the hearing screening are seen for the specialized testing necessary to determine how good their hearing really is. The 40+ percent who refer on the hearing screening and aren't seen for further testing might have permanent hearing loss. In fact, odds are that one in five will have hearing loss, and this one-in-five who referred on the hearing screening but didn't get follow-up testing will be missed and won't receive timely intervention. These babies might as well not had the hearing screening in the first place! One would expect when the baby becomes a toddler with speech delay, further evaluations will be explored, and a diagnosis and intervention will occur between the ages of two and three years (as was the case, historically, before Dr. Downs challenged the status quo in pediatric audiology). Efforts and funding toward improving follow-up testing for newborn-hearing-screening refers have determined a few reasons why babies who don't pass the screening are "lost to follow-up." The distance to travel to a qualified audiologist to perform the testing and follow-up care has been shown to be a reason some babies are lost to follow-up. Additionally, when mothers receive some form of state assistance (such as Medicaid or subsidized housing), or mom's native language is not English, chances go up that the baby is lost-to-follow-up. These children who are born into less economic opportunity are perhaps the most in need of timely diagnosis and intervention, as their family support network has less capacity to advocate for their needs. While increasing economic opportunity and access to English-language learning might be beyond the purview of the JCIH, increasing the number of pediatric audiologists qualified to provide the specialized testing for newborn hearing screening refers is an attainable goal in the near future. Efforts to increase access to qualified pediatric audiologists has received some successes in recent years, primarily through appropriate funding to government agencies, such as Maternal and Child Health (MCH), the National Institute on Deafness and other Communication Disorders (NIDCD, one of the National Institutes of Health), and the Centers for Disease Control and Prevention (CDC).

HOW IS HEARING TESTED IN INFANTS AND YOUNG CHILDREN?

If newborns and very young children can't reliably show us how good their hearing is, how is their hearing tested? Earlier in this chapter, the term "objective hearing test" was introduced. In reality, all hearing tests have elements of "objectivity" (just the facts) and "subjectivity" (a person's interpretation of those facts). The objective hearing tests are really tests that don't require the person being tested to actively participate. One "subjective" hearing test we all know is the fundamental way hearing is tested: raise your hand when you hear the beep. Most of us had this hearing test done in elementary school, or in our primary care doctor's office when we were children. This kind of "listen for the beeps" test has a fair amount of objective facts controlling how the test is done: the beeps are carefully controlled for the frequency (which our brains register as pitch) and intensity (which our brains register as loudness), and the person being tested raises his or her hand (the fact they give a response shows they admit to hearing the sound). But, this kind of test is a "behavioral hearing test," and requires the active participation of the person being tested. A person could choose to not participate (for instance, if he is trying to fake a hearing loss), or might not be able to participate (for instance, the instructions for how to respond are given in a language she doesn't speak and she doesn't understand what she is supposed to do). In pediatric audiology, we don't expect a child younger than five years old to be able to keep his or her attention long enough to reliably raise his or her hand in response to the tone on the "beep-test." Listening for soft beeps and raising your hand every time you hear them gets boring, quickly. Pediatric audiologists have developed techniques to teach children to give a reliable behavioral response to a sound they can hear by giving carefully timed rewards for correct responses (a technique psychologists define as "conditioning"). An experienced pediatric audiologist can condition a child as young as six to eight months of age to reliably respond to even the softest sounds they can hear. At younger than six to eight months, it is not expected a child can reliably participate.

Recall in chapter 1 and earlier in this chapter, one of the principles of JCIH's standard of care is to diagnose congenital hearing loss by age three months. Since the three-month-old can't be conditioned to give reliable behavioral responses, the pediatric audiologist uses objective test techniques to estimate what the child *would* show behaviorally, if the child were old enough to participate in a behavioral hearing test. Technology to objectively estimate hearing ability was developed in the late 1970s and through the 1980s, and made its way into mainstream pediatric audiology clinics in the 1990s (on the coattails of the JCIH 1994 position statement calling for objective hearing screen for all newborns). The two main tests that objectively estimate hearing are Auditory Brainstem Response (ABR)[6] and otoacoustic emissions (OAEs; pronounced "OH-TOE-acoostic E-missions").[7] ABR is a very special kind of electroencephalogram (EEG—brain wave measurement). The ABR is also called Brainstem Auditory Evoked Response (BAER) and Brainstem Auditory Evoked Potentials (BAEP) by certain medical professionals; these are all the same test, just a different name.

OAEs are tiny sounds created by the cochlea, and can be measured in the ear canal with very sensitive microphones; these sounds can be caused by playing carefully constructed sounds into the ear canal, and measuring what the cochlea sends back. If OAEs are present, it gives good evidence the cochlea is normal, or at least near-normal. The ABR measures tiny electrical signals from the auditory nerve and "nerve checkpoints" up the brainstem (which is the part of the brain that sits just above the spinal cord). Carefully constructed sounds played to the ear cause the nerves to "fire" (give off electricity), and the nerve firings can be recorded by sensors ("electrodes") placed on the head of the person being tested. If the sound can be heard, the nerves fire. If the sound can't be heard, the nerves don't fire. The readings presented on a computer screen to the audiologist are squiggly lines that have characteristics the audiologist has been trained to identify and interpret as true nerve responses. Hence, there is some subjectivity in performing the ABR; specifically, reading the ABR takes experience and mentoring before an audiologist can accurately conduct this test with confidence.

The good thing about the ABR and OAE signals is they don't require the active participation of the person being tested, and they don't hurt. But they do require *passive* participation; that is, these signals are so small that moving around wipes out the tiny electrical signal from the nerves when an ABR is being performed, and vocalizations (e.g., crying, squeals) wipe out the tiny OAE sounds from the cochlea. For this reason, these tests are usually done while the baby is asleep. In a baby under age six months, getting him or her to take a nap for an hour or more is a reasonable expectation as long as the timing of the test is reasonably close to the baby's naptime. The ABR test takes between forty-five minutes and ninety minutes, depending how quietly the baby sleeps during this time and how easy it is to zero in on the softest sound that causes the nerves to fire. The OAEs usually take only a few minutes, but these tell us only "good" or "not so good" cochleas, and don't tell us exactly how loud sounds have to be made for the baby to hear. The ABR is more valuable for estimating true hearing sensitivity, so quite often the audiologist opts to do the ABR first and save the OAEs for the end. The two tests complement each other, with the results of the two taken together to help explain how good hearing is, and if something needs to be done to help the baby's access to communication. These two tests together as well are used to document if the type of hearing loss is actually ANSD. While not so common, it is necessary to look for ANSD in a child with hearing loss, as the recommendations and expectations are different if the hearing loss is due to a problem with the cochlea (sensorineural loss) compared to a problem with the connection to the nerve (ANSD).

There is a third objective test that is done nearly every time a child is seen for any kind of hearing testing: a test called tympanometry (pronounced "TEM-pan-ahm-etry").[8] This test takes only a few seconds (and also doesn't hurt: it feels a little like a finger in the ear), and the person being tested can be awake, but should not be vocalizing (it's very hard to get a good tympanometry measure on a screaming child, so the audiologist may have to repeat it over and over to catch a few seconds between cries). Tympanometry tells us if the eardrum and middle ear bones (the ossicles) are moving as they should. If they are not moving, then there is suspicion of a blockage (like fluid in the middle ear) contributing to any existing hearing loss. If there is fluid, we would expect there to be a mild hearing loss (at most, a moderate hearing loss) and we would expect it to be temporary. If tympanometry results suggest there is fluid, but the degree of hearing loss measured by ABR is more like a severe-to-profound hearing loss, then perhaps hearing will be better when the middle ear is clear, but it's unlikely hearing will be all the way back up to normal. This is an example why the diagnosis of hearing loss is often a process, rather than an event. If there is fluid present on top of an underlying congenital sensorineural hearing loss, it may be unclear how severe is the permanent hearing loss until the fluid clears. Another reason the diagnosis is sometimes a process, not an event: the baby wakes up before the testing is completed and won't go back to sleep. This would require another "sleep hearing test" appointment to try to complete the testing.

As long as the baby sleeps for some of the testing, it is likely at least some information about the baby's hearing will be known. Adequate time for sharing of the information, and processing that information, needs to be set aside at the end of the test. This time spent in counseling is supposed to be part of the appointment, but sometimes counseling ends up hurried because testing ran long and another family is there for their scheduled appointment. This can make counseling feel rushed, and can interfere with some of the most important exchange between the audiologist and the parent. In cases where counseling time is limited, it is reasonable to keep the amount of information shared, and processing the meaning of this information, to a minimum, and schedule another in-person or telephone meeting with the audiologist. Even if there is adequate counseling time, a follow-up phone call the next day or two is very helpful, especially if permanent hearing loss was diagnosed. Experienced pediatric audiologists know that when hearing loss is diagnosed, it is normal and expected for the parent to have powerful emotions, which need to be given appropriate space and respect. Quick access to the audiologist for clarification and emotional support is beneficial to both the parent and the audiologist.

The objective hearing tests described so far—ABR, OAEs, and tympanometry—are fundamental to testing newborns and very young children, but are not the only tests available, or the only ones that should be done. Which tests to do, and when, depends on the questions that need to be answered. When permanent hearing loss is confirmed in a young baby (for instance, by three months of age), interventions should start immediately, and another set of tests should occur about every three months for the first year, unless there is a strong reason to monitor the hearing more often, or less often. Why check hearing every three months? Often, the degree of hearing loss doesn't change, but it does change often enough (roughly one-third to one-half of all hearing losses progressively worsen). If hearing does change, it might have a big impact on choosing the appropriate interventions. If there is strong suspicion for rapid progression of the hearing loss, repeat testing might happen more often than once every three months. If the degree of hearing loss is in the severe-to-profound range (with normal tympanometry), it might be that any progression (worsening) of the hearing loss won't have a significant impact on the plan to provide the child with meaningful access to language—so, it might not be necessary to repeat testing so often. If the hearing loss wasn't fully characterized in the first appointment (as it often is not), the next set of tests should occur quite soon (ideally, within a week or so, if there are no other extenuating circumstances that interfere with this happening). Which tests should be performed, and how often, should be for specific reasons to guide the interventions, and not just for the sake of following a clinical protocol. If there are any questions regarding the necessity of another appointment, another set of tests, and so on, you (the parent) should ask for justification. In today's healthcare arena, all too often tests are conducted out of habit, or to satisfy that no test was left undone, rather than because it makes sense for guiding the family along their path. Many times, these tests (while covered by health insurance) apply first to a deductible (the amount of money each year the family is responsible to pay, according to their specific health insurance plan, before health insurance kicks in). Kids are expensive: ask questions about the necessity of further testing. Healthcare providers sometimes need to be reminded to work efficiently on the family's behalf.

After roughly one year of monitoring hearing about every three months, if the permanent hearing loss has not worsened, it is reasonable to lessen how often tests are repeated to roughly every six months. If there is suspicion of a change in hearing, however, repeat testing should occur within weeks. As the baby grows older, it is less likely the baby will sleep easily in the strange environment of the audiology clinic. Often, after a baby is six months old, the likelihood of timing the tests during a solid nap is much more uncertain than before the baby is six months old. Often, in children with suspected or confirmed sensorineural hearing loss who needed repeat testing after the age of six months (but before they can reliably show us how good their hearing is, behaviorally), testing is conducted while the child is under sedation or anesthesia. It is possible the clinic can conduct testing under light sedation, if they have adequate medical staff and the young child is very healthy. If there are any concerns about the baby being able to be safely sedated, facilities often opt to test the child under general anesthesia, with a pediatric anesthesiologist providing specialized medical support during the procedure. Some hospitals require there be present a surgeon of record (such as an ENT surgeon) who has overall responsibility for the patient's care. This ENT may or may not be directly involved in the evaluation and management of the hearing loss, but is an integral team member, as will be discussed in chapter 7.

Putting a child under general anesthesia may seem like going to extraordinary lengths just to test his or her hearing. Many children don't need this, thankfully. For instance, if hearing loss is confirmed by several different types of tests (say, at age three months and six months), and an intervention plan is put into place before the child is six months old, the next time hearing needs to be tested is at nine months of age. Most typically developing nine-month-olds can show us how good their hearing is through behavioral hearing tests that are conducted in special sound treated rooms with calibrated earphones and loudspeakers. That is, nine-month-old babies can sit up (typically on a parent's lap) and be conditioned (taught) by the pediatric audiologist to turn their head to look for music, speech, and warbled or hissing noises, even if those noises drop down very close to the softest sound they can hear (i.e., their threshold of hearing sensitivity). We all naturally turn and look where a sound comes from when that sound is new, obvious, and it's not yet clear how important that sound is: is it a good thing or a bad thing that sound just happened? Is that sound meaningless, so I don't need to pay attention to it?

When a sound is new and obvious, our instinct is to check it out to see if it is important (was that noise downstairs someone breaking into the house?). It's a reflex: babies do this too, and reflexively turn to a sound when it's played. The more speech-like the sound is (like music, mother's voice, a cartoon character's voice) the more likely they will alert to it. When the child alerts and turns to the sound, the audiologist turns on an animated puppet or turns on a short cartoon clip on a screen to reward the child for turning toward the sound. The child may start looking around to find the puppet or cartoon again after the sound is turned off, but the audiologist waits until the child is looking away, and presents the sound again (a sound that is again expected to get the child to turn his or her head). If the child turns toward the sound again, he or she gets the visual reward of seeing the puppet light up and dance, or the short cartoon clip. In most children between about eight months and twenty-four months, two or three presentations of an interesting sound with a well-timed visual reward is enough to teach the infant or young toddler the listening game. A well-conditioned child can maintain attention to the game for easily fifteen to twenty minutes, and respond at or near his threshold of hearing. That is, if a child is sufficiently motivated by the reward (getting to see the puppet or cartoon), she turns her head as soon as the sound is audible. She doesn't wait until the sound is loud enough that she is certain she hears it. This type of behavioral hearing test is called Visual Reinforcement Audiometry (VRA), and it is usually highly entertaining for the parents, too, the first couple times they participate in it.

When a child is between age two and three years, the puppet and cartoon clip becomes less interesting, and his motivation to participate in VRA drops pretty quickly. A hearing test technique that is suitable for three- to five-year-olds (and some two- to three-year-olds if they are mature) is called Conditioned Play Audiometry (CPA). Once children are able to follow two-step commands (which is about the time they are ready to be introduced to potty-training), their brains become a bit too sophisticated to be entertained by the puppet/cartoon clip in VRA. They are able to follow the rules of simple games, and they understand the concept of "winning" a game. Capitalizing on this developing brain, the audiologist has the child sit in the sound-treated room and teaches him a listening game (either sitting in his own chair, or on the parent's lap). Here's an example: the child is sitting, holding a block, and either an audiology assistant or the parent holds a bucket while sitting across from the child. The audiologist says over the loudspeakers or ear-phones, "Put it in!" at a level that should be easy for the child to hear. Even if the child doesn't have the language to understand "put it in," he can get the gist of the game by the assistant or parent cuing him to drop the block in the bucket. The audiologist doesn't even need to say actual words: she can say "bah-bah-bah" and the child is visually instructed to drop the block in the bucket. After a couple practice rounds, three- to five-year-olds catch on, and sometimes really get into the competition of it! The more motivated they are, the more likely they are to stay focused for the necessary testing time (fifteen to twenty minutes) and the more likely to respond (that is, put the block in the bucket or peg in the pegboard) at levels at, or close to, their threshold of hearing. Be-tween ages two and three years, VRA is too young for them, but CPA might be too old . . . children between ages two and three years (espe-cially boys, in my experience) catch onto the rules (wait, listen, and *then* do it!) but are too impulsive to wait for the sound to come on before dropping the block in the bucket. Sometimes it just takes patience and reinstruction, and sometimes it's necessary to come back on another day to complete the testing.

HOW ARE HEARING TEST RESULTS DOCUMENTED?

The underlying purpose of all tests, whether they are objective tests or behavioral tests, is to get a clear picture of the type of hearing loss (conductive, sensorineural, or both, meaning the hearing loss is "mixed"), the degree of the hearing loss (mild, moderate, severe, or profound), and what the degree of hearing loss is across the pitch range most important for hearing and understanding speech. Hearing test results are usually plotted on a graph called an audiogram (figure 3.1). On this graph is plotted the softest sounds that are heard, for the right and left ear, and using headphones, headbands, and/or loudspeakers to test the different parts of the ear. There are lots of different symbols used to describe what part of the ear was being tested, and these are shown in the audiogram symbol legend (figure 3.2). Speaking with many parents of children with hearing loss, most have said it is very helpful to learn what the audiogram means. Most audiologists are all too happy to teach parents (and kids as they get older), so don't hesitate to ask.

The audiogram is a graph of hearing sensitivity (reported in decibels, or "dB" for short; usually also specified as "decibels hearing level," or "dB HL") at the different frequencies (reported in Hertz, or "Hz" for short). The intensity scale (that is, loudness) is vertical, with the softest sounds (-10 dB, -5 dB, 0 dB, etc.) at the top and the loudest sounds (100 dB, 105 dB, 110 dB, etc.) at the bottom. The further down the threshold of hearing, the more severe the hearing loss. The frequency scale (that is, pitch) is horizontal, from the lower pitches (bass sounds) on the left side (250 Hz, 500 Hz) the mid-pitches in the middle (1000 Hz, 2000 Hz), and the higher pitches (treble sounds) to the right (4000 Hz, 8000 Hz).

On the audiogram, sounds that are softer than the threshold of hearing would fall above the symbol and can't be heard. Sounds that are louder than the threshold of hearing would fall below the threshold symbol on the audiogram (and would be heard). If we take all the sounds of speech (vowel and consonant sounds) and measure their frequency and intensity (that is, their pitch and loudness), and plot them on the audiogram, it creates a banana-like shape (see figure 3.3). In this Speech and Familiar Sounds Audiogram is also the rough pitch and loudness of individual sounds of speech. You'll notice many of the vowel sounds and some of the low-pitch consonant sounds (like "m," "d," and "b") are on the left side, and are louder than the highest pitch consonant sounds ("f," "s," and "th") that are on the right side of the graph.

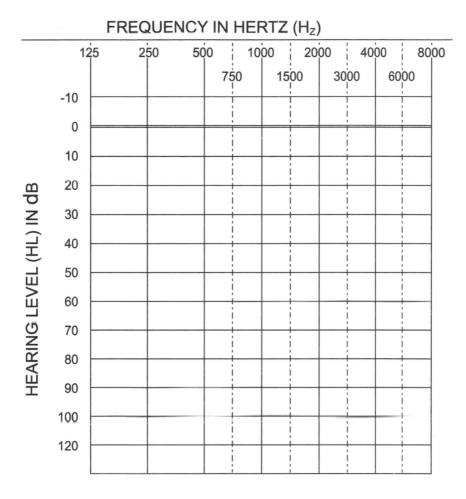

Figure 3.1.   Audiogram. The graph used to plot hearing sensitivity in decibels hearing level (dB HL) across the different frequencies (in Hz) important for hearing and understanding speech.

Very often, hearing loss is more mild in the low pitches, and more severe in the high pitches, so speech can be heard (that is, the low pitches are heard) but can't be understood (because of the loss of the high-pitch speech sounds). Other familiar sounds, like the beeping of a microwave oven, refrigerator, and whispering are also plotted on the audiogram at the frequency and intensity most representative of those sounds. Where the hearing threshold symbols fall on this graph, relative

| | AIR CONDUCTION | | BONE CONDUCTION | | SOUND FIELD | NO |
	UNMASKED	MASKED	UNMASKED	MASKED	(NOT EAR SPECIFIC)	RESPONSE
RIGHT	O	△	<	[		↙
LEFT	X	☐	>	]		↘
BOTH			∧		S	↓

Figure 3.2.   Audiogram legend. The symbols used to show the softest sound heard when sound was presented to different parts of the ear using different kinds of headphones, headbands, or loudspeakers. If there was no response, even when the sound was played the loudest the equipment can play it, an arrow indicating "No Response" is added to the symbol.

to these speech sounds and other familiar sounds, gives you some idea which sounds can and can't be heard.

Tools like figure 3.3 are intended to help give some understanding to an otherwise invisible condition. They can't capture all the nuances of communication, like talking with someone you know well versus someone you have just met, or talking with someone closer versus further away, or with background noise present. Hearing tests that are intended to document hearing sensitivity don't explain what we actually do with our ears. We seldom listen for beeps and hissing noises at the threshold of hearing sensitivity. These sounds would be meaningless in our everyday lives. But these kinds of threshold tests (like ABR and behavioral audiometry) are done because in order to understand what was said, you have to be able to hear it in the first place. So, hearing threshold tests are a start (but not the finish) to figuring out how good, or not-so-good, a person's hearing is.

There are additional tests to further understand hearing abilities. The most often used are speech audiometry tests, which use carefully selected words or sentences presented at a level either at normal conversational speech (around 55 dB HL) or at a level the person can hear it better (for instance, presented at 75–80 dB HL for a person with a mild-to-moderate sensorineural hearing loss). Sometimes these tests are performed with background noise, to further characterize how well the person can hear when the listening environment is more challeng-

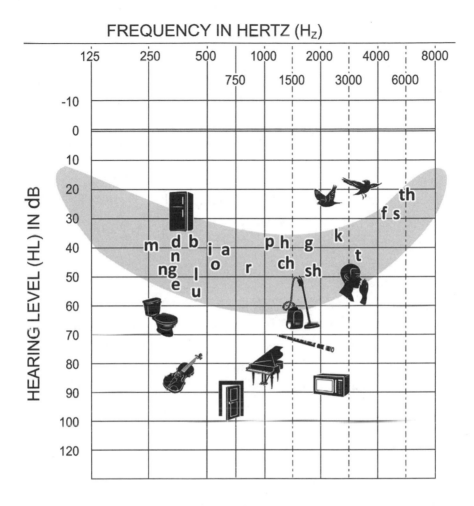

Figure 3.3.   Familiar sounds audiogram. An audiogram with the sounds of speech positioned at their relative frequency and intensity. The shaded area (the "banana") shows all speech sounds as they would fall on the audiogram. Familiar sounds usually are made up of lots of different pitches, but are plotted at the most representative frequency and intensity (pitch and loudness) on the audiogram.

ing than a perfectly quiet hearing test sound room. Two children with identical audiogram test results might do very different on tests of understanding speech in noise. How those two children are managed to improve communication access needs to reflect their specific needs, regardless what the audiogram shows. Children with ANSD are most significantly affected by the presence of background noise. Some can hear quite well when it is completely quiet, but may have no usable hearing when there is just a little background noise. Once a child with ANSD is old enough to participate in speech audiometry tests, his or her true hearing abilities can be much better characterized than the tests that only try to estimate hearing sensitivity.

Finally, tests of a person's ability to hear, understand, and remember sounds can be performed to characterize a person's auditory processing abilities. Auditory processing disorders are not as well defined as hearing loss due to problems with the ear (for instance, the middle ear or cochlea), but cluster under an umbrella of challenges that manifest as difficulty using speech for higher-level tasks, like learning or following directions. Auditory processing disorders are suspected if a child has at least normal intelligence, has normal language abilities, but is encountering great difficulty in school grasping new concepts. These kinds of tests purposely make the listening environment during the test very challenging by adding background noise or competing (background) words, to tap into how the brain organizes and makes sense of spoken instruction (for instance, a school teacher's lesson). If there is a problem with how the brain organizes what the ear hears, having a formal diagnosis and recommendations for school accommodations can make a huge difference in a child's academic success. For children with hearing loss, they tend to always do poorly on tests for auditory processing disorder. This is because the ear typically doesn't hear well enough (even with devices to maximize hearing, like hearing aids or cochlear implants) for the brain to make use of the sound when the listening environment is made challenging.

Hearing tests provide valuable information, which is necessary to figure out "what's next." But the tests themselves do not improve hearing; they are not therapeutic. It is rare, but in my career, I've seen babies who were screened over and over in the birth hospital because the hearing screening personnel did not understand the purpose of the screening (pass or refer only, not "fix"). It's even more rare, but it has happened, that children with "suspected" hearing loss have multiple ABRs in their first few months of life but results are deemed "inconclusive" because the squiggly lines of the ABR were not correctly interpreted. So, the test is repeated, which only serves to delay interventions. Hearing tests need to be performed adequately to help guide the intervention efforts, but no more than what is needed. It can be very difficult to get a complete hearing test in a child, either because you need the child to sleep soundly and he or she doesn't, or because the child is old enough for behavioral hearing tests but the audiologist can't adequately condition the child to give a hearing test that reliably reflects his or her hearing sensitivity. Repeat testing is necessary in such cases, and this is very common. But lack of complete tests results should never cause a full stop for introducing interventions, because the child's brain doesn't stop developing while we figure out just how good his or her hearing is. The experienced clinician uses all available information, however incomplete, to figure out "what's next."

On that note, in chapter 4 we'll delve deeply into understanding how hearing loss impacts the child, his or her access to spoken communication, the impact this has on social-emotional development, and the impact this has on the family.

4

THE IMPACT OF CHILDHOOD HEARING LOSS

In this chapter, we'll step through the way hearing is used by a child's brain to decode the pops, hums, and hisses of speech into something meaningful and useful. We'll diverge and consider what could happen if there is hearing loss (and it goes undetected) and the brain doesn't have a chance to figure out how to decode spoken language. The challenges can be widespread: from interfering with the way the brain is supposed to develop, to problems with self-esteem, to problems developing good relationships. In this chapter, we also consider the more subtle, but very consequential, impact of chronic ear infections and unilateral and high-frequency hearing loss. This chapter sets the stage for why it's necessary to check every newborn for hearing loss, and diagnose and manage it quickly. It's in some ways painting a reasonable "worst-case scenario," but based on what commonly happened when children were more often late-diagnosed. The challenges described in this chapter are what we work to overcome.

We take hearing for granted. Here are examples of sounds that are easily taken for granted, but easily lost: the "pssssss" from unscrewing the cap off a bottle of carbonated soda is an unmistakable sound. The crackle from pouring milk into a bowl of Rice Krispies is a sound many of us know from early childhood. The squeak of a swing on a playground is a happy memory for many of us from childhood. If you've spent a lot of time with toddlers, either a younger relative or your own children, you can probably think of some sounds that make them come running. For my twenty-three-month-old daughter, Emma, it's the sound of the ice dispenser from our refrigerator. She loves chewing on crushed ice, so she drops everything when she hears someone getting ice. The examples above (the soda bottle, Rice Krispies) are easily heard by someone with normal hearing, but not so for someone with a mild to moderate hearing loss. They have full experiences, of course, but different from people with normal hearing. Happy memories from childhood may have subtle differences for people with childhood hearing loss. The rich memory of the smell, sight, and sound of a campfire on a summer night may instead be a rich memory of the smell and sight of the campfire (without awareness there was a sound of crackling). Not hearing some of these everyday sounds, and experiencing all the sounds of the world that most people hear, has an influence on how a person gets to know his or her world.

Not hearing the more subtle sounds of speech has obvious and immediate consequences. Babies start saying their first words at roughly one year of age. But language-learning begins much earlier than one year: in order to figure out how to say a word, and that words in general have meaning, the baby has to overhear words thousands of times. Babies automatically (that is, reflexively) make sounds in the first few months of life. They cry when they are hungry or need comfort. They make gurgling noises as they discover the feeling this gives them in their mouth and throat, and play with these sounds. Parents reinforce the baby playing with sounds by making delighted sounds back at them, and talking directly to them in an animated voice. We do this animated voice (baby-talk, or "motherese") back to babies by instinct. We seem to be programmed to give babies the feedback they need to keep playing with their sounds, even from the earliest ages. As babies get older, they become more attentive to faces and movement around them, and show a preference for the face and voice of their mother. Babies start to babble with purpose, rather than just making sounds randomly. As babies continue to hear people around them talking, their babbling gets more sophisticated. Instead of "babababa" and "dadadada" they start to vary the consonant sounds: "badadadababada." They change the pitch of their voice to make it go higher or lower (or both) while they are babbling. They figure out how to make more and more consonant sounds in their babbling, and learn good control of their lips, tongue, and breathing. When a baby blows a raspberry for the first time, it tickles her lips, and parents laugh and delight, so the baby does it again. But it takes amazing coordination to make the lips pull tight around the tongue, but make the tongue relaxed enough, while blowing out enough air to make it vibrate loudly. Some babies learn to make an incredibly loud, high-pitched shriek, which they think is funny, but everyone else in the house grimaces and covers their ears. Babies will see this reaction in their family, and do it again, because it's fun to make other people do things with your voice! A baby figuring out that his or her voice influences other people's behavior is an extremely important milestone in early language development. [1]

As babies get closer to saying their first words, their varied babbling takes on a rhythm that actually sounds like words. The babble is paced like a real sentence, with inflection in the tone, and with the baby pausing to breathe where the grown-ups normally do (at the end of a phrase or sentence). And at some point, something clicks in the language area of the baby's brain, and the baby says "baba" to refer to his or her bottle, and the baby keeps referring to the bottle as "baba" and only uses that word for bottle. And shortly after, "dada" may come along. "Mama" might come along first, but the "m" sound is harder to make than the "d" sound so oftentimes "dada" is said before "mama" (sorry, moms). Even though these earliest words aren't really said correctly, the parent understands them, and so does the baby. This mutual understanding of the baby's spoken language is a huge milestone in the baby's language development. Over the next few months, the number of words the baby learns to use consistently increases: from only a few, to around twenty within a couple months, to fifty to a hundred within a couple months after that. Around age two years, toddlers have hundreds of words (or word approximations), and they figure out they can put two words together in a simple phrase: "more milk" or "mama go." These simple phrases are strong evidence another language milestone has been achieved, and the child is off to a lifetime of language learning.

This normal acquisition of spoken language happens because the parts of the brain that are involved in *thought*, and turning thoughts into language, receive input from the part of the brain that receives sound from the ear. Thought and language work so closely together that it's near impossible to consider what a thought actually is without some "symbol" (for instance, a word, or a sign) to give it meaning. The part of the brain responsible for making vocal sounds (controlling the mouth and tongue and vocal cords, etc.), was told to make these sounds by the thought and the language centers of the brain. The sounds that are produced by the throat and mouth are heard by the ear, which sends the sound to the hearing-part of the brain, which give input to the thought and language centers. There's a pretty complicated exchange between the different parts of the brain, and the vocal sounds made and then heard. These different parts build on each other: the ear has been eavesdropping on parents who make lots and lots of different sounds with their voices, and the thought and language centers tell the speech-producing centers of the brain to make the mouth-throat (etc.) imitate those sounds. The baby's vocalizations are really simple, and the baby keeps practicing to make the imitation more precise. It also feels good to make the sounds, and the grown-ups usually like it when the sounds are made, so the baby has great motivation to keep going. As time goes on, these systems (as well as quite a few other areas of the brain, including vision, sense of touch, smell, etc.) come together to give the baby a sense of where he or she is in the world, and who he or she is in it, including the relationships that are important to the baby (for instance, parents and siblings). This "sense of self" is an extremely important *cognitive* milestone.[2]

Lots of toddlers are speech delayed. I've understood from speech-language pathology colleagues that as many as 10 percent of all eighteen-month-olds are delayed in their speech development and may need speech-language therapy to help promote their speech development.

Often, the underlying root is these children are still trying to figure out how to coordinate the mouth, vocal cords, and breathing (which really is a pretty complicated thing to do), and with the right kind of therapy, they can come along pretty well. Some truly do "outgrow" their speech delay without any intervention. Some have challenges with the way their thought-centers communicate with the language centers. When, and how, intervention for these speech-language challenges should be sought is outside the perspective of this book, but suffice it to say: learning to talk is really complicated. It takes a lot of practice, and a lot of good input right from the earliest days of life. It takes brain systems that are communicating well, and a home environment that gives the child good motivation to engage verbally.

HOW DOES HEARING LOSS IMPACT SPEECH AND LANGUAGE?

When hearing loss is present, that "good input right from the earliest days of life" is interrupted.[3] Depending how much hearing loss is present (and what kind), maybe some everyday sounds and speech sounds are heard while others are not; maybe no sounds, except the loudest, like a siren or door slam, are heard.[4] Babies with hearing loss do cry, gurgle, and play with the sounds their voice can make. They might change the pitch and loudness of their voice too. When there is significant hearing loss (moderately-severe or greater), babies tend to babble only vowel sounds (these vibrate, and feel good), and likely they can hear some of these sounds from adults (at least, when they are close), and they very likely can hear the sounds when they make them.[5]

The underlying meaning of words spoken to them (the "symbol" of the thought being communicated) might be lost on them, though. For instance, the word "milk" means a white liquid that feels good to drink and relieves the pain in the belly called "hunger." The sounds that make up the word "milk" have nothing to do with the white liquid that feels good to drink. But when the brain hears all those sounds and sends those to the language centers, those sounds are decoded and when the word "milk" is said, the baby is able to think of what that word symbolizes (something he or she wants). So what if the sounds of the word "milk" don't all come through? When only a few speech sounds are heard by the ear with hearing loss, lots of words with different meanings (and sound different to people with normal hearing) sound a lot alike to the baby with hearing loss. There is no clearly defined symbol for the white liquid that feels good to drink. As the baby's thought-centers grow more and more mature, he might do so without the benefit of the language centers helping to formulate distinct symbols for each different thought. Because the language centers aren't instructing the speech-producing centers to continue to practice making lots of different sounds to imitate the grown-ups (likely because the baby doesn't know there are different sounds to make, or to be imitated), the baby doesn't make meaningful progress in speech-language development. This delay in making good progress in speech-language development as a result of hearing loss means there is a lack of understanding between the child's attempts to share thoughts with the trusted grown-up. The child's sense of self is at risk. The child's ability to construct more complex thoughts, and express those (which is necessary for seeing which trusted grown-up will meet the child's needs, thereby establishing relationships) is at risk. The disconnect in communication that interferes with shared understanding between the child and the rest of the family means the child with hearing loss and speech-language delay cannot understand, and cannot be understood. But he or she still has the same wants and needs of a child with normal hearing and normal language, and if these wants and needs aren't met, the child will find alternative ways to get them. Which usually means challenging behavior.

Parents dread days when their toddler misses a nap. Young children need routines that include a solid nap during the day, so they have the energy to navigate their world during waking hours. When a nap is missed, that energy is depleted, and you have a cranky toddler on your hands. Cranky toddlers don't have the patience to problem-solve when they don't get their way. They don't have the motivation to try to negotiate different ways to get what they want. They either get what they want (and sometimes the parent just doesn't know what that is, and the child doesn't have it in them to communicate it), or they fall to the floor thrashing and shrieking. There is no consoling them at this point. There is no redirecting them to better behavior. It's game over; whatever you were doing (or wanted to do), that's over.

A child who cannot express wants or needs effectively, due to a barrier being able to communicate the complex thoughts and needs swirling around in his or her head, has two choices: try really hard to make the other person understand you by any means you have (like gesturing, leading, pointing, etc.), or throw a tantrum. If the earlier attempts to communicate wants and needs are not understood, the tantrum becomes the only remaining option. The tantrum might not be very effective at getting what the child wanted originally, but it is an expression of the frustration that has built up due to the inability of the child to make himself or herself understood. It must be very scary for a child who needs something, and can't count on anyone being able to decipher what it is they need. It makes complete sense that the child would have a tantrum, just as a release from the frustration that easily builds up. Over time, the child's patience for trying to be understood grows very short, and he or she is very quick to exhibit challenging behavior. What does the child have to lose? Nothing else works anyway.

The anger, fear, and frustration that accompany an inability to understand, and be understood, compromises the child's social-emotional development. When the child's sense of self is one based on isolation from others in the family, it is easy to understand why that child might feel like an outsider. Children model their relationships with peers and other adults based on their relationships with family members. If their relationships with family members are challenged due to the communication barriers, they will not have had the opportunity to learn how to make friends with peers, or negotiate relationships with non-family-member adults. Easily adjusting to an expanding social circle (which happens when the child goes to preschool or kindergarten) is an impossibility. Children without the social skills necessary to form relationships with new peers are challenged to find a way to be incorporated into the group. If the child isn't successful making friends, and is an outsider from the social circle, it is reasonable the child's self-esteem will be negatively impacted.

When a child's language is delayed because of a lack of awareness of the varied sounds of speech that means the child would not readily understand the different letters of the alphabet are associated with different speech sounds.[6] Learning to read and write (that is, developing literacy) depends on the child having a large vocabulary and understanding each word is a symbol for something unique. Breaking those words into each sound, and assigning a letter of the alphabet to those sounds, is the beginning of literacy. Future success in school and in work depends on the child making good progress in literacy throughout his education. With good reading and writing skills comes further ways to explore and expand thoughts, which is another important milestone in cognitive development. A child who is a successful reader no longer is restricted to learn from only those people immediately around her: if he or she can read a book, she can learn from someone she has never met (the author). Her access to a broad range of ideas, which stimulate her own, is limited only by her language maturity.

Successes in academics and in making friends improves a child's self-esteem, and helps the child navigate relationships at home. Each member of the family has a place within the family unit, and the relationships are built upon past experiences and current expectations. If a child has learned to negotiate his place at school with peers, this can help that child negotiate challenges with older or younger siblings who compete for the parent's attention, or access to the television. For a child who has limited language due to hearing loss, that child's place in the family might be as an outsider, perhaps with one (or both) parents taking primary responsibility for meeting the child's needs. Rather than sharing in the parent's attention across siblings, the child with hearing loss might need to monopolize the parent, leaving siblings to have less time with the parent. This would reasonably breed resentment in the siblings, and feelings of guilt in both the parent and the child with hearing loss.

Thankfully, these are only hypothetical risks, explained in the extreme case that the hearing loss goes undetected for a long time, and no intervention is given until well into grade school. It would be tragic for a child who is bright and friendly to have an undiagnosed hearing loss that results in untapped abilities, with the child never having the opportunity to reach his full potential, academically, occupationally, or socially. The efforts to diagnose and then manage hearing loss centers on addressing these risks, which are a real threat to the child reaching her full potential.

So far in this chapter, we've explored the potential impact of significant permanent hearing loss in both ears across the speech frequencies. It's safe to say the descriptions above are broad generalizations, and certainly don't apply to all children born with hearing loss, even those who aren't found until they are toddlers. But there are common themes that serve as take-home messages: the ear is how the brain accesses sound, including speech. Speech is the common form of language for those of us in the hearing world, which is made up of "chunks of thought" (symbols). The give and take of these chunks of thought start very simply, and grow to be more complex as the brain matures. As the brain decodes the speech into language, the brain's ability to form more complex thoughts accelerates. Language becomes a tool for the brain to make itself smarter. At the same time, the exchange of language between the growing child and caregiver is a foundation of relationship-building in the family. When there is hearing loss, and it's enough that the only speech sounds heard are a garbled string of vowel sounds without decipherable meaning, speech doesn't get translated by the brain into language. Without a foundation in language, the child is limited in his or her ability to build relationships. It's a good thing, then, that we look for hearing loss in all children (at least in the developed world), and have interventions that are effective at getting language going quickly.

As we've discussed at length, not all hearing loss is the same. How does temporary hearing loss affect speech and language development? How is speech and language impacted when the hearing loss only affects the very high pitches (for instance, those speech sounds like "f" and "th," as in the words "first" and "thirst")? Is speech or language affected by one-sided ("unilateral") hearing loss? These are great questions that have been the subject of debate in the scientific and medical community for a long time, and there isn't total agreement. We'll take each one in turn.

Almost all children get at least one ear infection in their lives. The prime time for a child to get an ear infection is between ages eighteen months and two and a half years, but some children get ear infections regularly when they are in grade school.[7] And, of course, it usually comes on in the middle of the night, with the child waking up, wailing and inconsolable. While the child is sick, she is very uncomfortable, with the fever and ear pain, but she recovers, good as new, most of the time. In maybe 10 percent of toddlers, ear infections just keep coming back, time after time. It's possible that between bouts of true infection (when there is fever and obvious signs), there is fluid lingering in the middle ear that isn't causing pain or fever, but is acting like an earplug. When hearing is muffled, and the child is literally "hearing underwater," a lot of speech sounds aren't making it through. Those sounds that do happen when the talker is close by (like when reading a book at bedtime), or when a parent comes closer and raises his or her voice to stop the toddler from doing something he knows he shouldn't (like color on the walls or climb up the pantry shelves). At a normal distance, when the child is playing over in a corner while the grown-ups are talking, instead of eavesdropping on the conversation and giving the language centers some really juicy input, the child is floating in his own little underwater world, unaware there is good language stimulation happening only ten feet away. It's no surprise that children with chronic middle-ear fluid seem to not be paying attention, are easily distractible, and often get into trouble for "not using their listening ears."

In the roughly 10 percent of kids who have fluid that persists three months or longer, there is concern that they are missing out on enough language-learning time that they might be speech-delayed. While most kids with chronic ear infections do develop speech on time, there is enough evidence to comfortably say that, all things being equal, if a child has fluid in the ears for months at a time it can affect how well he or she picks up spoken language. The evidence is less solid, but there is suspicion that chronic ear infections as a toddler is associated with auditory processing problems when the child is older. Perhaps the change in hearing, from good to not-so-good as the fluid comes and goes, interferes with the child's brain making sense of the world, how to attend to important information and exclude unimportant background noise, figure out where sounds come from, and the like.

Sometimes children have very good hearing sensitivity through the low to middle frequencies, but have high-frequency (only) hearing loss. Imagine on the audiogram with speech sounds and familiar sounds (figure 3.3) good hearing from the low frequency side (250 Hz, 500 Hz) through the middle frequencies (1000 Hz, 2000 Hz), but hearing drops off at 3000 Hz, 4000 Hz, 6000 Hz and 8000 Hz. This is pretty common in children who were very ill as newborns and received powerful intravenous (IV) antibiotics to save them,[8] or have gone through chemotherapy to treat cancer.[9] Children with high-frequency hearing loss usually develop speech and language very well, but they miss subtle things,[10] like the "t" sound at the end of a word that makes it past-tense: "walk" vs. "walked." They just don't hear the "-ed" at the end of the word: "I'm going to *walk* to the store. Do you want to come?" The next day: "We don't need to drive. I *walk* there yesterday." Missing out on that marker for past tense is just one example. Using an example from earlier in this chapter, what if the words "first" and "thirst" sounded exactly alike? For someone with high-frequency hearing loss, these two words are indistinguishable. Of course, those of us with a lifetime of language behind us would easily figure out which word was said ("first" or "thirst") in a conversation based on the context. But for a child just learning the meaning of these words, the inability to tell the difference based on how they sound creates confusion (which easily leads to frustration). Because of not hearing these high-pitched speech sounds, the child may have trouble learning to make these sounds, himself. The child with high-frequency hearing loss might have a distorted "s" sound (for instance, a "lisp") that requires speech-articulation therapy. The child may need language support to develop an awareness and understand the meaning of the missing "t" sound that means things happened in the past.

And it's not just these subtle high-pitched speech sounds that are affected: when rooms get noisy (like the typical classroom) and someone is talking about something important that you really should pay attention to (like, the teacher), it's not so easy to hear every word perfectly, because the background noise (and possibly echo, or reverberation, in the room) is interfering. Kids with normal hearing across the whole range are able to pick up on important speech cues here and there, and fill in the gaps caused by the interference. Kids with high-frequency hearing loss can't hear those random speech cues that make it through the background noise and echo, so are at a disadvantage, compared to the other kids with normal hearing.[11] Often, they appear distracted, and it isn't as easy to get their attention as children with normal hearing. If the hearing loss is unknown, they might be labeled as having problems with attention and following directions; unfortunately, a question of hearing loss is almost never first on people's minds when concerned about why this particular child isn't as "focused" as he or she should be in class.

There are some similarities between the problems faced by children with high-frequency hearing loss and children with unilateral hearing loss. It used to be that we expected that if a child had normal hearing in at least one ear, he or she had all the hearing necessary to do just fine. But we are born with two ears for a reason. Our two ears work together to help us figure out where things are around us. Our two ears give us directional hearing, which is incredibly important for safety (which way is that car coming from?). Our two ears help us hear the person who is in front of us, while damping down other conversations that are to our sides or behind us. This "hear the person in front of you better" is something called "The Cocktail Party Effect."[12] Our two ears zoom in on the person in front to help us hear better, even when the background noise is pretty loud. If a person has no usable hearing in one ear, but hears well in the other, he doesn't have the ability to zoom in on the person in front of him and suppress the background sound, since all sound seems to be coming from the side of his hearing ear. He also doesn't tell direction of sound nearly as well. This matters to children most when they are in a classroom, where the teacher is at some distance from the child with hearing loss and the side conversations, paper rustling, noisy heating/air-conditioning system, LCD projector, and so on, create background noise. These children also seem to be easily distracted, it's harder to get their attention, and they often miss directions spoken by a teacher. Children with unilateral hearing loss are at a disadvantage compared to the other kids with normal hearing in both ears. Sound familiar?

The challenges with high-frequency hearing loss in both ears and unilateral hearing loss are very similar, and most obvious when children are in school. Before school, most children with high-frequency hearing loss or unilateral hearing loss develop speech and language relatively on time. There may be some subtle problems (for instance, difficulty learning to use "s" and past-tense) but these are easily overlooked if the hearing loss is unknown. Hearing most certainly wouldn't be the most obvious reason for these subtle problems. The most groundbreaking research in the areas of unilateral and high-frequency hearing loss has been conducted by Drs. Fred Bess and Anne Marie Tharpe at Vanderbilt University in Nashville, Tennessee.[13] In a landmark study headed by Dr. Bess, researchers looked at school performance (grades, whether or not they had to repeat a school year, and teacher ratings) of third graders, sixth graders, and ninth graders, and tested their hearing after-the-fact. The researchers compared how children found to have normal hearing did to how children found to have unilateral hearing loss or bilateral high-frequency hearing loss did. On average, 3 percent of kids with normal hearing had to repeat a grade by the time they were in ninth grade. Thirty-seven percent of kids with unilateral or high-frequency hearing loss had to repeat a grade by the time they were in ninth grade. Teachers were asked to fill out screening questionnaires about their students' academic performance, and across the board, for the children with these subtle (previously undiagnosed) hearing losses, teachers judged their reading comprehension, language skills, spelling, and even science knowledge to be poorer than kids with normal hearing.

We can make some safe bets that those kids with undiagnosed, subtle, hearing loss had poorer self-esteem than their normal-hearing peers. Doing badly in school and labeled as the "inattentive" or "problem" student means adults will grow to have expectations of the child struggling, and quite often, the child meets those expectations. It's easy to miss that hearing loss was the most significant reason for the problems in school. When a child struggles and adults have low expectations, and inappropriately blame the child for not doing better, it is no surprise there is a high rate of high-school drop-out in children with subtle hearing loss. This, of course, has enormous consequences on their future employment opportunities: all because a unilateral or high-frequency hearing loss wasn't picked up and addressed from the earliest ages.

Thankfully, due to the excellent work by Drs. Bess and Tharpe and others, and the responsiveness of schools to identify and address problems like this, the severe negative consequences described above happen less often than they used to. School hearing screenings are pretty good at catching these subtle hearing losses, and once the child is seen for full audiological and medical evaluation, educational supports can be put in place quickly.

5

HOW IS HEARING LOSS TREATED?

This is a long chapter that covers a lot of detailed information. It includes a brief introduction to surgical and medical treatment of conductive hearing loss and gives a more in-depth review of treatment for permanent hearing loss through the use of devices, like hearing aids and cochlear implants. Since people who use hearing aids and cochlear implants (CIs) still struggle to hear well in background noise, assistive listening devices (like FM systems) are invaluable to improve ease of listening. Why these are helpful, and when they are most important to use, is included in this chapter. Finally, we take a brief look at what the future holds with regard to curing deafness through medications or stem cells. Impressive technological strides have made it much better for people with hearing loss than any time in human history. But there's still a ways to go to make hearing loss less of a barrier.

If a consequence of hearing loss is isolation (from family, friends, and the rest of the "hearing" world) then treatments to help hearing are supposed to reduce the isolation. Most treatments do not actually cure the hearing loss. If there is a temporary form of hearing loss that can be treated medically (medication or surgery), it is usually a very simple form of hearing loss (albeit, often a very big deal when the hearing loss is present). It is possible that within our children's lifetime, there will be some therapy that can cure "permanent" deafness, through stem cell transplants, gene therapy, or some other way to make the damaged system repair itself. For now, with permanent hearing loss, if a family believes that hearing should be a significant part of their child's experience, then it is imperative to fit the child with the right devices to help his or her hearing.

WHAT TYPES OF HEARING LOSS CAN BE TREATED WITH MEDICINE OR SURGERY?

In chapter 2, we talked about ear infections and the mild conductive hearing loss these cause. Most often, this type of hearing loss is temporary, since hearing gets better when the ear infection is treated and the fluid inside the middle ear clears up. Most of the time, the ear infection either clears up on its own, or is cleared up by a course of antibiotics. If the fluid and infection are persistent, the child's primary care doctor may refer the child to an Ear, Nose, and Throat (ENT) surgeon. The ENT doctor may recommend surgical placement of tiny tubes ("tympanostomy" or "PE" tubes) in the child's eardrum. When placement of PE tubes is recommended, it is done in an operating room with an anesthesiologist putting the child to sleep under general anesthesia. Once the child is safely asleep, the ENT surgeon looks down the ear canal using an operating microscope and uses a tiny knife to make a small cut in the eardrum. If fluid is present in the middle ear (as is almost always the case when tubes are needed), the surgeon uses a small suction tube to suck out the fluid. This is sort of like sucking mucous out of the nose of a child too young to blow his own nose. That might sound gross, but when it's needed it makes them breathe *much* easier. When fluid is suctioned out of the middle ear, it means hearing improves just as quickly. After the fluid is suctioned, the surgeon carefully slips the PE tube into the hole they made in the eardrum. The eardrum heals very quickly (within hours) *around* the outside of the tube, leaving the hole in the tube open to allow air from the ear canal to pass into the middle ear (and vice versa). Keeping the middle ear well ventilated helps the middle ear stay healthy. It doesn't eliminate the possibility of an ear infection, but it reduces the number of ear infections while the tubes are in. The most common type of PE tube stays in the ear an average of eight to eighteen months, and is eventually pushed out by the eardrum growing over behind the tube, forcing it out of the eardrum and into the ear canal. Eventually, the tube comes out of the ear canal on its own in the child's earwax.

Other types of hearing loss that are medically or surgically treatable are much less common than ear infections. They do happen though. Some of these other causes of hearing loss are problems with how the bones of the middle ear were formed while the baby was developing in the womb, how the ear canal was formed (that is, if it stayed closed and didn't open before birth), and other ear health problems that are rare but have very serious health consequences (like cholesteatoma and mastoiditis). Each of these more rare but serious ear problems often require both ENT surgical intervention to manage the ear health problems, as well as audiological intervention along the way to help with the hearing loss specifically.

It can happen that some types of sensorineural hearing loss can change rapidly (sometimes temporarily, sometimes permanently). If this happens, the audiologist gets the child to an ENT quickly to be evaluated for whether or not it makes sense to go on a course of steroids to try to rescue hearing. This type of hearing loss, "sudden sensorineural hearing loss," might be totally unexpected, or might be anticipated because of the underlying cause of the hearing loss. Some reasons this might be expected is if the child is known to have a temporal bone malformation (like "enlarged vestibular aqueduct") or a history of certain infections that can cause sensorineural hearing loss (like congenital CMV or meningitis). Steroids reduce inflammation, which is a natural reaction of the body's immune system to the injury, but inflammation often causes problems on its own. If inflammation is the cause of the hearing loss, and the steroids are given quickly enough, they might reduce the inflammation in the inner ear and some (or all) of the hearing that dropped might come back.

WHAT TYPES OF HEARING LOSS CAN'T BE TREATED WITH MEDICINE OR SURGERY?

Generally speaking, hearing loss related to the inner ear or hearing nerve are not medically or surgically treatable. These include sensorineural hearing loss and auditory neuropathy spectrum disorder (ANSD). Recall from chapter 2 that lots of different things cause sensorineural hearing loss. When the inner ear is affected by genetics, the baby being born extremely premature with breathing problems, injured by a side effect of powerful medications, or damaged by an infection, the delicate cells that are responsible for giving us sensitive hearing die off and don't get replaced. This makes the hearing loss permanent. Think of a spinal cord injury: if the spinal cord is cut, the severed ends heals over with scar tissue, but the ends don't connect, and the person loses the ability to control parts of the body that are below where the spinal cord injury occurred. Someday, we may be able to regrow the spinal cord nerves and "cure" paralysis caused by these kinds of injuries. But not yet. We'll take a brief look into the future in this chapter about the kinds of things that might happen, down the road, to regrow these delicate cells in our inner ear in the hopes of restoring hearing.

Also later in this chapter, we'll review CIs, which do have a surgical component to the management of sensorineural hearing loss and ANSD; however, the surgery is part of giving the child the device to give them a sense of hearing, rather than to actually correct the underlying physical issue in the ear. So, surgery for CIs is not considered "treating" the hearing loss itself.

HEARING AIDS: PERSONAL AMPLIFICATION

If the child has a permanent hearing loss, and the family believes that hearing should be a part of the child's experience, then she will need some type of device to help her hear better. These devices (hearing aids, CI, other devices like the Baha, etc.) maximize the use of the remaining hearing system. What does that mean, "maximize the use" of the hearing the child has left? It means *selectively* making some sounds louder, or even adjusting the pitch (the frequency) of important sounds if there is little to no hearing left in that important pitch range. It is true, hearing aids often just "make sounds louder," but it is the way they selectively do this that makes them exquisitely sophisticated devices! Hearing aids are now computer programmable, and selectively boost the sounds that are too soft to hear up into the range where the child *does* have hearing.[1] Alternatively, they can shift the frequency of sounds (usually the very high-pitched sounds) to a lower register where there is better hearing. And they do this while letting those louder (audible) sounds through without boosting them too much. In fact, for really loud sounds, the hearing aids actually drop those sounds down, so the really loud sounds are not uncomfortable. Essentially, hearing aids that are programmed correctly act as a prosthetic device, taking over what the inner ear would have otherwise done if there were no hearing loss. Recall from chapter 2, people with sensorineural hearing loss hear the louder (audible) sounds just as loud as people with normal hearing. But sounds that fall below their hearing thresholds simply don't exist. Correctly programmed hearing aids take those sounds that are below hearing threshold and boost them up into the *residual* hearing range. This "residual hearing range" is the range of sounds from the softest you can hear to the loudest you can tolerate. For a person with normal hearing, this range is big (easily 100–110 decibels). For a person with hearing loss, this range is much smaller: for example, a person with a moderate hearing loss may be able to hear sound starting at 60 decibels ("dB"), and the loudest tolerable is 110 dB. This residual hearing range, then, is 60–110 dB (or, only 50 dB residual hearing range, rather than 100 dB for the person with normal hearing). Sounds below that hearing threshold (in this example of moderate hearing loss: 60 dB) have to be boosted by the hearing aids somewhere above 60 dB in order to be heard. But the sounds that are already above 60 dB can't be boosted by the hearing aids by the same amount, because: (1) They don't need to be; and (2) There's not that much range left to take such a big boost. So, a soft sound might be boosted up 30–40 dB, and a moderately loud sound might be boosted 10 dB. Very loud sound might be *dropped* by 5 dB.

Hearing aids "squish" sounds into the person's residual auditory range as best they can. The greater the degree of hearing loss, the less range (residual hearing area) is available. So, some soft sounds end up being lost if the hearing loss is moderately-severe or greater, even with well-programmed hearing aids. When sound is "squished" it doesn't sound quite the same as it does to a person with normal hearing. Since vowel sounds ("a, o, e," etc.) tend to be louder than consonant sounds (e.g., "s, th, p, k," etc.), but consonant sounds carry the information necessary to understand the word, hearing aids boost sounds in the mid to higher pitches (consonant sounds) more than low pitches (vowel sounds). There are some reasonably good examples of hearing with hearing aids available on the web and other resources. A few examples of using well-programmed hearing aids to manage common degrees of sensorineural hearing loss are on my practice's website (www.bosaudconsul.com). It's much easier to hear what someone is saying when the consonant sounds are boosted, but speech sometimes loses its "warmth" (which often comes from a good balance between low and high pitches). There are trade-offs. Do hearing aids work? Yes. Research has demonstrated that children identified with hearing loss by three months of age, and are fitted with hearing aids within one month of diagnosis (and at the latest, by six months of age) end up doing as well academically and socially as their normal-hearing peers.[2] A very touching video was pointed to me by a parent of a child with hearing loss: it's accessible via YouTube, and is a video of a little boy (Lachlan) who is fitted with a hearing aid when he's seven weeks old.[3] He fusses when the snug earmold is inserted into his ear (as expected), but then his facial expression changes as his audiologist and his mother talk. At the time of this writing, this video can be accessed at: https://www.youtube.com/watch?v=T05oyzahoLY. A Google search for "Lachlan's first hearing aid" will likely provide a link if the one listed here is out of date.

Hearing-aid technology in the 1980s and before was very limited. Hearing aids didn't sound very good, and they did little more than make all sounds louder. This helps in a quiet room when a person with at least a moderate degree of sensorineural hearing loss (or any degree of conductive hearing loss) is in a one-on-one conversation. But with 1980s technology, as soon as background noise is present (which is pretty common), they are of little use. Being forced to talk with someone only when there is no background noise is quite limiting (that is, isolating).

Thank goodness that with the advent of computer chips and advanced digital signal processing, hearing aids have gotten much smarter. As well, the hearing-aid microphones have advanced to the point they can zero-in on only what is directly in front of the listener, or even direct their focus to voices to either side. An example when this either-side listening might be helpful: listening to someone beside you in the car when both of you are facing forward. A ton of work has been done in hearing aid technology over the past couple decades to make hearing aids work better in noisy situations. While they don't "fix" the hearing loss, they work much better than they used to. How many people are still using a computer running Windows 1995, or dial-up Internet access? Hearing-aid technology has harnessed the rapid advances in computer processing to make hearing in all environments easier. CIs have benefited as well from advances in computer technology, as well as from advances in hearing aids. If something works well in hearing aids (for instance, directional microphones), then these improvements often translate into CIs.

What hearing aid is the right kind of hearing aid for a child with permanent hearing loss? Almost always, a "behind-the-ear" (BTE) hearing aid gives the best performance (works better) to meet hearing needs. BTE hearing aids sit on top of, and behind, the outer ear (specifically, the pinna) and a tube runs from the sound output speaker in the hearing aid down into the ear canal. Because a child's ear grows pretty rapidly until the age of twelve (and really fast in the first two years of life), it is necessary to replace the earmold that fits into the ear and ear canal when the old one is too small to fit well. Could a child use hearing aids that fit entirely in the ear, or down in the ear canal, with no parts that fit behind the ear? Yes . . . but the outer shell of the hearing aid would have to be remade as the ear grows. This gets expensive to replace the shell, and while the hearing aid is being remade, the child is "off the air." Quite simply, in-the-ear hearing aids aren't a good option for children, at least not until their ears stops growing as fast (near the teenage years). An alternative that might be a reasonable compromise is a "receiver-in-the-canal" (RIC, also called RITE) device, which still has a part sitting behind the ear, but the part that goes down into the ear canal is a tiny wire. A custom-made earmold for a RIC hearing aid is still a good idea for children (for lots of reasons, including making sure the hearing aid stays in the ear), and then only this earmold would need to be replaced. It used to be that RIC hearing aids weren't strong enough to be used by people with greater than a moderate degree of hearing loss, but they have gotten better. Now many people with severe sensorineural hearing loss can use RIC hearing aids, if they use a custom earmold.

It is very important that the earmold fits snug and fits well in the child's ear, and parents become really good at putting the earmold in fast. Think of a custom-made pair of shoes: if made right, they should fit great! If not made well, or the shoe isn't put on all the way and the heel sticks out, you can get a blister or they may fall off. Earmolds need to be snug in a person's ear so that the sound can be kept in the ear. When earmolds don't fit very well, sound can leak out. When this happens, the hearing aid often squeals (this is called "acoustic feedback" or just "feedback"). When the hearing aid is squealing, the sound is not going into the ear. It's not dangerously loud for the child, but sound isn't going in like it's supposed to. Likely, the child doesn't even hear the squeal (but everyone else around does).

Keeping hearing aids in a child's ear is not always easy. Early on, young babies just let things happen (after a little fussing). Putting on clothes sometimes makes young babies fuss, but usually they tolerate clothes once dressing is done. My twenty-three-month-old daughter, Emma, is going through a "naked" phase: after getting her dressed, she loves to pull off every last stitch of clothes (starting with her socks). In the car seat, her shoes and socks come off almost immediately. Toddlers with hearing aids very often go through similar phases of expressing their independence. What's a parent to do? Pick and choose your battles. Sometimes it's right to put the hearing aids/clothes/diaper right back on. Sometimes it really doesn't matter. During listening activities, it should be an expectation that hearing aids stay on (because that's how the child hears best). When it's cold outside, it's an expectation the toddler keeps his or her coat and gloves on. It becomes a battle of wills, sometimes. As all parents do, you just do your best! Other parents of children who use hearing aids have gone through these challenges and often have great tricks. Your child's audiologist almost certainly has a number of tricks as well to keeping the child's hearing aids in place. The last chapter of this book includes helpful suggestions from parents who have "been there, done that."

Hearing aids are medical devices that can be extremely beneficial, making softer sounds audible while still keeping louder sounds tolerable, that is, as long as the professional fitting the hearing aids has the necessary education, training, and experience to work with young children and babies with hearing loss. Unlike older kids with hearing loss (older elementary-school age and up), young children and babies cannot report whether the sound is adequate and tolerable. While it is unlikely, it is possible for hearing aids to be fit to boost sound far too much, and risk damaging residual hearing further. More often, the hearing aids are set too softly and sound that could be made audible (loud enough, and therefore, useful) isn't boosted enough. This renders the hearing aids less effective than they should be for giving good access to spoken language. It is *imperative* that the person fitting the hearing aids have, at a minimum, an audiology degree (AuD or PhD, or another designator indicating the person is an audiologist), knowledge of best practices in pediatric hearing-aid fittings (the American Academy of Audiology has a comprehensive pediatric hearing-aid fitting protocol),[4] and objectively verify that the hearing aids are providing enough, but not too much, boost to sound. This "objective verification" is usually done with special equipment that includes a very thin and flexible tube that is inserted into the ear canal with the hearing aid in place. This very thin tube is connected to a microphone that is hung on the child's ear and can measure the sound coming through the hearing aid and into the ear. This way, the verification system can tell if the hearing aid is boosting sound just the right amount. This is the only way to know, for sure, that the hearing aid is programmed and working correctly, since the young child can't tell us. The best person to provide this kind of care is a pediatric audiologist. There are web-based resources to identify a qualified provider (for example, www.HowsYourHearing.org).

If a child has a sensorineural hearing loss, and also has ongoing ear infections, it is important the ear infections be treated very aggressively—more aggressively than you would for a child who doesn't have an underlying sensorineural hearing loss. The reason for this is that the child with sensorineural hearing loss already hears less than optimally when the ears are clear and hearing aids are in the ears and working great (remember, hearing aids help hearing, they don't cure the hearing loss). Any additional conductive hearing loss acts as an earplug, further reducing the residual hearing. As well, many older kids who use hearing aids will say they really don't like having an earmold in their ears when they have an ear infection. Not using hearing aids during an ear infection means the child is *really* off the air until the infection clears. As a result, it's typical for a young child with sensorineural hearing loss who has a few ear infections to get PE tubes faster than a child with normal hearing and occasional ear infections.

COCHLEAR IMPLANTS: WHEN HEARING NEEDS A BYPASS

When the degree of hearing loss is so severe that there is very little residual hearing range, hearing aids may not be able to provide good enough access to speech sounds. Children with severe or profound hearing loss typically fall into this category. Hearing aids can give good awareness of environmental sound, and might help the child with severe hearing loss know when someone is talking, but the child might not be able to understand what is said. When hearing loss is this significant, the hearing aids are not expected to support acquiring spoken language through hearing alone. Thankfully, there is technology that can take over when hearing loss is this severe: CIs. CIs are medical devices that bypass the severely damaged hearing system, and give direct electrical input to the hearing nerve. The CI has two main pieces: one part that is surgically implanted in the cochlea (inner ear) and under the scalp, and one part that is worn on the ear and head. See a photograph of the two parts of an implant in figure 5.1.

The part that is surgically implanted is the "receiver stimulator and electrode array." The electrode array is a bundle of wires and twelve to twenty-two electricity emitters (electrodes) that are very carefully inserted into the damaged cochlea by an ear surgeon. These wires are connected to an electronic component called the "receiver stimulator" that is placed under the skin of the scalp and controls how the electrodes deliver electricity to the hearing nerve. The externally worn parts include the external processor and microphone (together, these usually look like a large behind-the-ear hearing aid) connected to a wire with a magnet in a circle. See figure 5.3 for a photograph of a child wearing the external CI processor.

Several weeks after the surgery is performed to insert the internal parts into the cochlea and under the scalp, and the area has sufficiently healed, the external processor is programmed to give "initial stimulation" to the internal parts—this is the first time the child hears with the CI. The magnet (the part that is a circle and has a wire leading to it from the external processor) sits on the scalp directly over where the receiver stimulator is placed by the ear surgeon. This piece transmits commands across the thin skin layer of the scalp to the receiver stimulator, which tells the electrodes what to do.

The part that is responsible for making sense of the sounds of the world is the external processor. The external processor has microphones on it that zoom in on speech (much like hearing-aid directional microphones do). The sounds picked up by the microphones go to the elec-

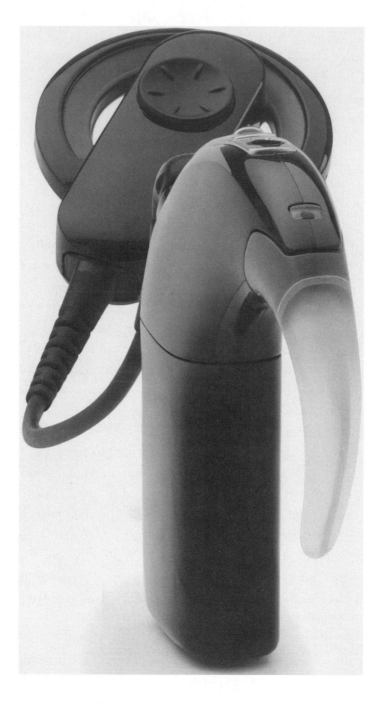

Figure 5.1.   Images of the external processor and internal receiver stimulator.
Picture provided courtesy of Cochlear Americas, © 2014 Cochlear Americas.

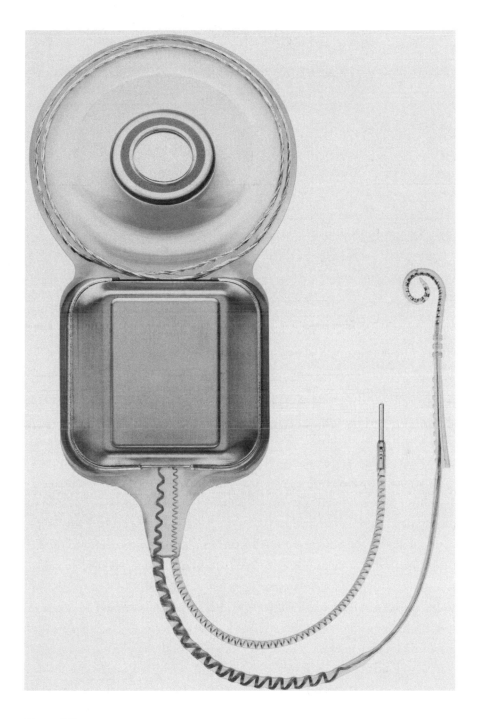

Figure 5.2.

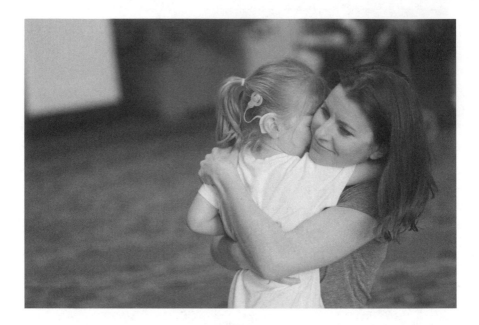

Figure 5.3.   A child with a CI wearing the external processor. Picture provided courtesy of Cochlear Americas, © 2014 Cochlear Americas.

tronic system in the external processor, where the sounds are broken down into discrete bits, with low-pitch through high-pitch sound separated out. These "chunks" of sound make up speech: depending on the CI system, there are as many as twelve to twenty-two discrete "chunks" that make up sound from low to high pitches.

These discrete chunks are assigned to stimulate the different electrodes that have been inserted into the cochlea. The hearing nerve is stimulated by the different electrodes in patterns, according to the CI program, and that signal is sent up to the brain to be decoded as something meaningful (for instance, language). The audiologist programming the external processor tests the child with the implant to see how much electricity needs to be sent to each electrode to be "heard," and how much electricity is "too much." It's essentially the same as figuring out how loud a sound has to be played to be heard, and how loud a sound is when it becomes uncomfortably loud. Only it's done with electricity instead of sound. But in truth, recall in chapter 2 that sound is *normally* turned into electrical signals by the cochlea, so all "sound" makes its way to the brain as electrical signals. So, the CI does something very similar to what the normally functioning ear would do: send electrical signals to the hearing nerve and on up to the brain where the decoding actually happens.

Based on how the audiologist programs the CI processor, the child's hearing nerve is signaled that different speech sounds were spoken. The pattern that the brain receives from the CI doesn't necessarily sound like real hearing; at least, not at first. But it does work, much of the time. It gives access to low to high pitched sounds, from soft to loud, that couldn't be given by a hearing aid when the hearing loss is severe or greater. Children who have very good outcomes often are able to hear most, or all, of the vowel and constant speech sounds.[5] Since they can hear these speech sounds so well, they often have very clear speech (clearer than if they heard only vowel sounds through powerful hearing aids).[6] In fact, there are many instances of a child with severe-to-profound hearing loss and a CI developing an accent particular to the region where they grow up. One example of a child with CIs acquiring a regional accent was pointed out to me by the parent of a child with CIs: This example can be found on YouTube at https://www.youtube.com/watch?v=fAtV-DctIeA.[7] In this video, two sisters living in Australia are age three years and four years. One has normal hearing and the other was born with severe-to-profound hearing loss and has a CI. Both have Australian accents. To an audiologist, this is amazing, because accents are a pretty subtle nuance of speech. The fact a CI *sometimes* gives good enough access to something so subtle is astounding. We wouldn't expect a regional accent to be picked up in his speech patterns by a child with severe or greater degree of hearing loss who uses hearing aids and communicates verbally. To be clear, though: if the hearing loss is less severe, and hearing aids are set correctly, it's likely the child will pick up the regional accent.

As hard as it might be to imagine what it sounds like to listen through hearing aids, imagining what it sounds like to hear through a CI is even harder. Rather than sounding a bit like listening over a telephone (hearing-aid simulations), CI simulations of listening to speech sound a bit robotic to a person with normal hearing.[8] There are some good CI simulations available on the web, but bear in mind that these simulations aren't exactly what a CI sounds like. These simulations are meant to give people with normal hearing an idea how hard, or easy, it is to hear and understand using a CI (not necessarily mimicking the sound quality). How children react when a CI is first turned on ("initial stimulation") is different from one child to the next. Sometimes, the new sound appears to be scary. They may get very wide-eyed and snuggle into their parent. Other children may find the new sound exciting! When children have their initial stimulation, different noise makers (like a xylophone, drum, tambourine, etc.) are available for them to experience how these sound through their CI. When they are excited by the new sound, they eagerly bang on the instruments, delighted by the new game: "Hey, when I hit this mallet on different bars on the xylophone, it makes different sounds!"

An amazing example that brought me to tears is a YouTube video of a teenage girl who seems to have modest expectations of the quality of sound from her new CI: https://www.youtube.com/watch?v=0B8Zj62LoUg.[9] Based on the content of this video, I'm surmising this teenager used hearing aids when she was younger, and already has a CI in her right ear; the video shows the initial programming and initial stimulation of the new CI in her left ear. This young lady's audiologist, who appears in the video, tearfully celebrating the joy of hearing with the young lady, is my mentor, Dr. Marilyn Neault, the Director of Habilitative Audiology at Boston Children's Hospital. It's people like Dr. Neault who represent the best of hearing healthcare. She is the audiologist who taught me the most about the importance of a family-centered approach to management of childhood hearing loss.

When a child gets a CI, whether they previously heard well with hearing aids or not, they need intensive hearing and speech-language therapy to learn how to hear with the CI (even if it sounds "really good"). Essentially, the brain has to be taught how to decode the patterns that the CI gives to the hearing nerve. It is reasonable to expect several hours per week of listening and spoken-language therapy sessions for years after getting a CI. The CI doesn't restore hearing, and what is heard through the CI doesn't necessarily come through as meaningful sound right away. Sometimes, it's a while before the brain decodes the CI input as meaningful sound. Is it easier than parents learning American Sign Language (ASL) and then teaching their child ASL? That's hard to say: both are a tremendous amount of work. The question becomes more "how would you like your child to communicate?" In the words of a parent of a child with CIs who also became proficient in ASL, "There is no way of getting out of 'work' when it comes to a parent teaching a deaf child language."

It is very important that parents have reasonable expectations about what hearing aids and CIs can do: they help the child to hear better. They do not guarantee good speech and language development, or good access to spoken language. Depending on the degree of the hearing loss, and how well a CI can stimulate the hearing nerve, the child may be able to hear lots of speech and environmental sound well. On the other hand, he or she may have limited hearing, even with the best CI mapping. Since CI requires surgery and extensive therapy for a long time to learn to use sound coming through the CI, it is extremely important that parents understand that a CI does not guarantee good hearing. How well a child does with a CI depends in large part on family support and the child's innate drive to use hearing to make sense of his or her world.[10] It is for this reason that it is important that parents considering CI for their child step through a candidacy process, learning about the risks and benefits of CI from a team who will provide a realistic perspective. Most children who use CIs *do* learn to talk, and they wouldn't have learned to talk (at least, not as early, or as well) if they didn't get CIs. But some children do not learn to talk, despite having CIs, and gravitate toward ASL. Responsible CI clinicians will advise parents of a child with profound sensorineural hearing loss that there is a possibility of the child learning to talk, but only with intense therapy and a lot of work.

WHICH IS BETTER: CIS OR HEARING AIDS?

All things being equal, when the hearing loss is severe or greater, CI gives a clearer sound than hearing aids do, after the brain "ramps up" to make sense of the signals from the CIs. If the degree of hearing loss is mild to moderately severe, it is likely hearing aids would do better than CIs (again, all things being equal, such as parent support, child's innate drive to communicate, etc.). Children who get CIs are, by and large, given a lot of speech and language therapy and auditory-listening therapy sessions. Children with hearing aids often don't get that same level of support, and the reason why has always baffled me. Do children with CI do better simply because they are more often enrolled in highly structured therapy programs, whereas children with hearing aids are not? Maybe. Learning to hear with technology (CIs or hearing aids) is a process, not an event.

DOES IT MATTER IF A CHILD HAS ONE HEARING AID OR CI, OR TWO?

It used to be that many children with hearing loss in both ears only got one hearing aid. The same was true with CI: all it takes to hear speech is one ear, right? That kind of thinking ("one is good enough") is decades old now. Recall from chapter 2 that we use our two ears together to make sense of our world ("where did that sound come from?") and to pick out the person we want to listen to in a crowd (the "cocktail party effect"). Most people with hearing loss in both ears report that having two hearing aids, or two CIs (or, a CI in one ear and hearing aid in the other) is better than having a device in only one ear. Two devices don't help as much as having normal hearing in both ears, but they are a big improvement in figuring out where sounds come from ("localization") and hearing in noisy environments. If a person has two devices, rather than just one, they won't be limited to making sure people sit on their "device side" in order to hear them better. It is less likely they will be surprised by someone walking up to them from their "unaided" side if they have two devices (they won't have an "unaided side" then). People have described having two devices makes them feel more confident and less anxious. Sometimes, though, it doesn't make sense to use a device on one side; for instance, if there's no residual hearing at all on one side, or for some reason the person isn't a candidate for a CI on the poorer side. In this case, the person with hearing loss in both ears, but can only use one device, is at a disadvantage. As a general rule of thumb, if two devices would be helpful, two should be used.

ASSISTIVE TECHNOLOGY TO IMPROVE UPON HEARING AIDS AND CIS

While hearing aids and CIs provide better access to speech and environmental sounds, when background noise is present, it can be hard for a person using such technology to hear. Even smart microphones that zoom in on speech can only help so much. The challenge created by background noise increases as the talker moves further away. This is most obvious in classrooms. It is shockingly hard to hear in the classrooms of mainstream public schools for a person with *normal* hearing. From the noisy heating/air-conditioning systems, to side conversations and paper rustling, to the teacher moving among students (that is, moving closer to a particular student, and then further away), classrooms are not easy listening environments. For a student with hearing loss, hearing aids and CIs aren't good enough to consistently hear the teacher.[11] Very often, it is recommended the student sit close to where the teacher usually stands ("preferential classroom seating"). But if the teacher moves among the class, as is typical, then preferential seating doesn't help that much.

An excellent solution is for the teacher to wear a microphone that picks up the teacher's voice and sends it directly to the student's hearing aids or CIs. This kind of system is called an "FM system" because the teacher's voice is transmitted to the child's devices by low-powered FM radio waves. The FM system is made of a microphone and wireless transmitter (usually about the size of a belt-worn pager) and the FM signal is picked up by special "boots" connected to the hearing aids or CIs. The benefit is obvious and vital: regardless how close or far the teacher is to the student with hearing loss, the child can hear the teacher as though he or she is standing next to the child the whole time.[12] Provision of the FM system is generally part of the school's obligation to provide the student with "equal access to public education," that is, the school is financially responsible for providing an FM system that works with the student's devices. We'll talk in detail about special education and Individualized Education Plans in chapter 7. For sake of the current discussion, it is important to understand that classrooms are challenging listening environments, and more is needed than hearing aids or CIs to hear well enough to learn.

Other assistive listening devices (ALDs) that work with hearing aids or CIs include "infrared" (IR) systems, "induction-loop" ("loop") systems, and Bluetooth connectivity. Many public places, like government buildings, are required by law to offer ALDs and display a message of their availability. IR systems are more common in theaters and are available upon request. Many concert venues, government buildings, and conference rooms have loop systems installed. Bluetooth is becoming more readily available, and hearing aids can be "paired" to Bluetooth-compatible devices (like car stereo, television, and smartphones like Android and iPhone). Each of these technologies follows a similar purpose: to bring the source of the sound (movie soundtrack, guest speaker, or caller) closer to the person with hearing loss. Using ALDs can make listening *much* easier, and so it's much more likely people with hearing loss will enjoy themselves, rather than struggling just to keep up.

WHAT ABOUT A CHILD WITH NORMAL HEARING IN ONE EAR, AND HEARING LOSS IN THE OTHER?

Should a child with hearing loss in only one ear (that is, a "unilateral" hearing loss) use a hearing aid or CI in that ear? Recall from above (and chapter 2), we use our two ears to make sense of the world around us and to focus on hearing what we want to when there's background noise. People with unilateral hearing loss often do well one on one in a quiet room, but struggle more in noisier environments than people with normal hearing in both ears would. And since hearing aids don't make hearing normal, the amount of benefit from using a hearing aid in this case varies. It also depends how much residual hearing is left in the poorer-hearing ear. If the hearing loss is to a greater degree than moderately severe, the amplified sound from the hearing aid may actual be heard by the other, normal-hearing ear before the ear with the hearing aid! That could create some confusion, although it could actually still be helpful; it might make them feel like they have less of a blank spot on their poorer-hearing side. Many people with normal hearing in one ear and hearing loss in the other strongly prefer having a hearing aid in their poorer ear: it can give a better sense of directionality, they don't get surprised as easily if someone walks up to them on their poorer-hearing side, and they feel more confident (and less anxious). Others find the sound through a hearing aid to their poorer-hearing ear distracting, and possibly making it *harder* to understand someone talking, than if they didn't use a hearing aid on that side at all. In the case of one-sided hearing loss, it's a matter of personal preference. If there is adequate residual hearing that a hearing aid might be of benefit, it's a good idea to at least give it a try.

While a child with good hearing in just one ear is expected to hear well enough to learn how to talk, once the child begins elementary school, it gets much harder for that child to keep up with normal-hearing peers. Whether or not such children use a hearing aid, they will need to use an FM system to help them hear the teacher better. While the use of a hearing aid is a matter of personal preference for children with unilateral hearing loss, it is imperative they use an FM system in the classroom. Several studies have shown that children with unilateral hearing loss who don't receive any interventions or educational support do much worse in school than their peers with normal hearing in both ears. They have to repeat grades at an extremely high rate, are often labeled as "inattentive" or "daydreamers," and do not perform as well on standardized tests. Consequently, kids with unilateral hearing loss often have the same social-emotional challenges as children with (untreated) hearing loss in both ears. When adequate educational supports are in place from early on, they do just as well, on average, as their peers who hear well in both ears.

For children with severe-to-profound hearing loss in one ear, and normal hearing in the other, a hearing aid on the poorer-hearing side might to be of limited benefit. The better-hearing ear would pick up the sound coming from the hearing aid before the ear with the loss, and it may be helpful, but it may also be distracting. Currently in the United States, it is not approved by the Food and Drug Administration (FDA) to provide a CI to a person with unilateral hearing loss. As a consequence, health insurance companies don't provide coverage. However, outside the United States, people with profound unilateral hearing loss do receive a CI and the reports suggest they do benefit. One high-profile recipient is Malala Yousafzai, who was nearly killed in 2012 by the Pakistan Taliban because she was targeted for her vocal advocacy for the education of girls in her country. As a result of her injuries, she has profound sensorineural hearing loss on the left side, and received a CI in that ear roughly four months after the attack. Perhaps someday, there will be adequate data supporting improved quality of life for a person with profound unilateral hearing loss receiving a CI, and the FDA will approve this indication.

In chapter 2, ANSD was described as a hearing disorder where the cochlea is working (at least relatively well) but the connection between the cochlea and the hearing nerve isn't working very well. Until not many years ago, it was considered categorically *wrong* to fit a person with ANSD with hearing aids; it was assumed they wouldn't do any good, since hearing aids are intended to enhance residual cochlear hearing. After some benefits were seen in the few people with ANSD who tried hearing aids, the use of hearing aids was recommended, but to program the amount of amplification to be conservative: don't give very much boost. As we learned more, it has become clear that people with ANSD don't always benefit from hearing aids, but if they do, they do better when the hearing aids are programmed according to their audiogram (that is, the hearing thresholds documented from a hearing test). Often, a person with ANSD does not get as much benefit from hearing aids as someone with a sensorineural (cochlear) hearing loss, even if these two people have very similar hearing thresholds (that is, their audiogram looks the same). If the person with ANSD gets very little benefit from hearing aids, CI is an option. If the child with ANSD isn't making good progress in spoken language, despite the family supporting this mode of communication and best efforts have been made to help the child's hearing through hearing aids and FM systems, then a CI should be considered. Assuming the child is medically a candidate for CI (for instance, is healthy enough and radiology studies, like MRI, show there's actually a hearing nerve present), then the benefit from CI is expected to be the same for a child with ANSD as a child with severe-to-profound cochlear hearing loss.

BAHA: BONE-ANCHORED OSSEOINTEGRATED DEVICES

Another kind of device is also available for children with permanent conductive hearing loss in both ears, or hearing loss in just one ear. a bone-anchored hearing system (often referred to as a "Baha" because it used to be called a "bone-anchored hearing aid"). The name of this system was changed because the term "hearing aid" created problems getting insurance companies to cover the cost of the device and related surgical and audiological services (historically, insurance companies don't cover the cost of hearing aids!). Sound can be delivered to the inner ear (cochlea) through the bones of the head: hold a tuning fork in your teeth or behind your ear and it's obvious. Bone-anchored hearing systems take advantage of this fact to help people hear when they have permanent conductive hearing loss, and they can't otherwise use hearing aids that go in the ear. If a person doesn't have ears or ear canals, conventional hearing aids can't be used.

Bone-anchored hearing systems include a very small titanium screw that is surgically implanted into one of the bones of the skull above and behind the ear by an ENT surgeon. Connected to the top of this tita-nium screw is an "abutment" that juts out through the skin of the scalp. About three months after the surgery to implant the titanium screw, the bone heals around the implant enough that the implant is now osseoin-tegrated (fused into the bones of the skull). An externally worn sound processor attaches to the abutment; this sound processor has a micro-phone and the electronics for processing sound, which is programmed by an audiologist. Instead of the sound being sent through the ear canal to the eardrum as with conventional hearing aids, the sound is sent through the bones of the skull to the cochlea where the sound is heard.

While the FDA has approved the surgery for bone-anchored hearing systems in children five years and up, the age at which a child can have the titanium screw implanted varies, and depends on how each child's skull is forming. If the skull is too thin where the screw needs to be implanted, the child isn't a candidate (yet . . . maybe she will be as she gets older). Regardless of the age when the surgery can be performed to implant the screw, these bone-anchored hearing systems can be mounted onto a soft headband (a "softband") with the external sound processor held against the skull. The sound processor sends the sound vibrations through the skull where they are picked up by the cochlea, in much the same way it would if it were mounted onto the abutment of an osseointegrated screw. Some of the downside to the sound processor being mounted onto a softband is that the range from softest to loudest sound that can be delivered is smaller, and the range of pitches that can be delivered isn't as broad as when the processor is mounted onto an osseointegrated post and abutment. While these are most useful in children with permanent conductive hearing loss in both ears, some people do use a bone-anchored hearing system if they have profound unilateral hearing loss. Just as with hearing aids and CIs, background noise creates a challenge for listening, and an FM system should be connected to help in the classroom.

WHO PAYS FOR THESE DEVICES?

Right or wrong, historically, hearing aids for children have not been covered by health insurance plans. CIs are almost always covered, but may require a lengthy "prior authorization" review process. The same is true with bone-anchored hearing systems: they are often covered by health insurance with prior authorization (now that they don't have the words "hearing aid" in their name!). Very few health insurance plans provide financial support (a "benefit") for hearing aids for adults, and by extension, hearing aids for children have historically been excluded as well. Through legislative advocacy in individual states, there are laws in twenty states (at the time of this writing) that mandate health insurance plans provide some form of financial benefit toward covering the costs of hearing aids and related audiological services.[13] While it is unfortunate that so many adults with hearing loss do not seek audiological treatment for treatable hearing loss, many do compensate with varying degrees of success, given a lifetime of language learning behind them. For children, time is of the essence! There is no acceptable amount of delay in proceeding with hearing-aid fitting. In fact, how fast a child is fitted with hearing aids is part of the standard-of-care mandates set down by the JCIII (2007) position statement. Once a child is identified with permanent hearing loss, hearing aids need to be fitted within one month (even if more testing continues to hash out the details of the hearing loss).

Whether or not your state has a law mandating some form of hearing-aid benefit in health insurance plans, it's important to find out, specifically, what your health insurance plan will and will not cover. Many health insurance plans will consider covering hearing aids and related audiological services, even if it's not automatically covered as part of the plan. Ask for a "prior authorization for coverage" to be considered, or ask about your policy's "appeals process." You may be surprised that you will qualify for at least some coverage. If you do end up not having insurance coverage for hearing aids, there are options for financial assistance. Some programs to cover costs for this type of treatment are based on family income, while others are not. Some local philanthropic organizations (such as Lions Club, Knights of Columbus, and Optimist Club) as well as state agencies (such as state vocational rehabilitation services) offer financial support. If financial support is possible, but causes a delay in getting hearing aids, many hearing-aid loan programs exist that can provide loaner hearing aids until financial assistance comes through.

As you work through all the challenges of being a parent, with the added challenges that come with your child having hearing loss, figuring out how to pay for hearing aids should be the last of your worries. Unfortunately, oftentimes it comes front and center. Seek the assistance of your child's audiologist and pediatrician: often they are aware which organizations in your area can help, and what hoops need to be jumped through to apply for help. As you figure out the costs associated with getting hearing aids, make sure you know what is included in the initial upfront costs of the devices, and what is not. Some audiologists bundle together the cost of the hearing aids with their professional services, while others separate out the cost of the devices from the professional services. Regardless, there can be a lot of out-of-pocket expenses, not the least of which is the cost of replacement earmolds, batteries, time off work and school, parking, gas, and so on. If financial assistance is available to cover any of this, take it!

MINIMIZING RISK FOR FURTHER HEARING LOSS

When a child has hearing loss, any further decrease in hearing can result in significant decrease in ability to understand, even if the amount of the decrease in hearing seems relatively small. This is particularly true if the degree of hearing loss is in the moderate range. For instance, if a child with a 60 dB hearing loss has a 10 decibel reduction (to 70 dB), that relatively small decrease matters a lot more than if the child's hearing dropped from 30 dB to 40 dB IIL. When the hearing loss is already down between 50 and 65 dB HL, there is a decent amount of residual hearing, enough that we can expect the child to get good benefit from hearing aids. A few decibels of hearing matters a lot in this range, though. If the hearing loss is less severe, small reductions in hearing matter, but there's still quite a bit of residual hearing, and adjustments to the hearing aid output should do the trick to compensate for the shift in hearing. On the other end, if hearing starts in the severe-to-profound range and hearing drops another 10 dB, the impact might, or might not, be significant: it depends how much benefit the child was getting from hearing aids anyway, and such a decrease might make it more obvious that the child will get more benefit from CIs.

To minimize risk for further reduction in hearing, parents and children (when they are old enough to take responsibility) should minimize exposure to sustained noise levels that are above 85 decibels.[14] This is about how loud it is when you have to shout to someone (with normal hearing) about an arm's length away for the person to hear and understand you. While a child's hearing aids *should* limit any further boost to the noise, be mindful that sustained exposure can cause decrease in hearing over time. What is "sustained exposure?" A child whose summer job is mowing lawns, and uses a gas-powered lawn mower and leaf blower eight hours per day, five days per week, would be at risk for some small decrease in hearing after several months. When the noise isn't necessary to hear, it's best to use hearing protection. Some over-the-ear earmuffs may actually be big enough to allow the child to wear hearing aids under them. Alternatively, taking out the hearing aids and putting in earplugs can be effective at protecting hearing. Be aware, though, that a child with hearing loss who is using hearing protection is seriously reducing their auditory awareness. The hearing loss, background noise, and hearing protection all combined makes any auditory awareness virtually absent.

If a child is engaged in music, either listening or playing an instrument, this is highly encouraged! Music is one of the most joyful things we use our ears for. A child with hearing loss should use headphones/earbuds if he or she wants to, and should not be discouraged from using an iPod. But just like any child (normal hearing or no) it's important to limit listening level and duration of listening. One rule of thumb is to listen no higher than 80 percent of the maximum volume control for ninety minutes per day (or less) if a person is using the headphones that come with the music player.[15] This "80-for-90" rule was developed by one of my audiology PhD students, Cory Portnuff, AuD, PhD, and me, to offer easy-to-follow recommendations for safer listening levels using headphones. Dr. Portnuff and I also showed that earphones that are designed to block out the background noise (sound-isolating earphones) are very successful in helping people to moderate their listening level on their own, without needing to resort to level-limiting headphones. If parents do want that extra bit of safety for their child who likes to listen loud, consider the Ety-Kids® earphones, which limit the maximum level while still isolating against background noise (http:// www.etymotic.com/consumer/earphones/ek5.html). For even more peace of mind, this earphone can be fitted with a custom tip that blocks out the most background noise while keeping the earphone secure in the ear. Alternatively, children may want to listen to music through their hearing aids or CIs, and they can do so by connecting their music player to their FM or Bluetooth streaming device (like some remote controls, for instance). The audiologist can even work with the child to adjust the settings on a "music program" that boosts sound to where the child likes it, while limiting the output to a reasonable level.

There are certain medications that have side effects that can damage hearing, and these are classified as "ototoxic." The medications that carry the greatest risk for hearing damage are powerful antibiotics that are given when someone is very ill and hospitalized (aminoglycoside antibiotics), have significant kidney dysfunction or heart failure and need diuretics to reduce the amount of water retained in the body (loop-inhibiting diuretics), and certain chemotherapy drugs used to treat cancerous tumors (cisplatinum and carboplatinum).[16] When these drugs are needed, it can be life or death, and these drugs do wonders to save someone's life. That said, if a child has need for powerful medications, parents should ask if there are any drug side effects that include damage to hearing. It is possible that some alternative medications can be used that are equally effective at treating the disease. Some over-the-counter drugs that carry some small risk for ototoxicity include aspirin (in high doses) and other NSAID pain relievers. Ask the child's ENT physician if there is any question about the safety of taking a certain medication.

FUTURE DIRECTIONS

Very recently, the FDA approved the use of hybrid CI-hearing aid devices in adults (but not yet in children). In hybrid CI-hearing aids, there is both an array of electrodes stimulated by a receiver stimulator and external processor, as well as that selective boost of sounds in the same ear. Theoretically, this would be especially helpful in people who have a reasonable amount of residual hearing in the low pitches, but little or no hearing in the higher pitches. The CI portion of this hybrid device would take over the job of picking up the higher pitches, while the hearing aid portion of the device would boost lower pitch sounds into the residual auditory area. This combination of technology is very exciting, and will help a large number of people whose hearing is just a little too good to go fully to a CI (and may want to keep some sense of acoustic hearing), but don't do all that well with hearing aids. As of this writing, hybrid CI-hearing aid devices are very new on the scene for adults. Often, the surgery to get the hybrid implant causes further damage to the region that has "aidable" hearing; that is, the hearing gets worse because of the insertion of the short electrode array of the hybrid device into the cochlea. If hearing drops too far, the patient may not be a candidate for the hybrid CI-hearing aid anymore, and would need a conventional CI instead.

Researchers who seek to find different ways to improve hearing in people with hearing loss have looked at a number of different pharmaceutical approaches to fix the underlying problems causing hearing loss. Since the 1990s, at least ten classes of drugs have been under development to lessen the impact of damage done to the cochlea by noise or certain medications.[17] Could we give a pill to people whose ears were injured that would rescue their hearing? What about using stem cells to regrow damaged sensory cells? If stem cells could be implanted in the cochlea of a person with hearing loss, could that person hear again? Could "gene therapy" be used to coax some of the surviving cells in a damaged cochlea to start growing into sensory cells (replacing ones that have been damaged)?

The answer to the questions above is "maybe, but not yet." The National Institute on Deafness and Other Communication Disorders (one of the National Institutes of Health) and many other government and philanthropic nongovernmental agencies have provided large amounts of grant funding to researchers trying to answer these questions with "yes."[18] It's clearly an extremely hard problem to solve.

The FDA requires extensive studies on drug safety first to see if the kind of drug can be tolerated, or if there are side effects that are just too dangerous. For instance, it's necessary to figure out if a new medication is safe and effective when trying to rescue hearing in a child who has hearing loss because he or she was born prematurely and has breathing problems. If a drug is found that can be safely tolerated, the next step is finding a drug that can be safely tolerated that actually works. This is even more of a needle in a haystack. What if the reason for the damage to the cochlea is from medication used to treat a life-threatening infection? Would a hearing-rescue drug interfere with the medication's ability to fight the infection? A good example of the worry over "treatment-interference" is chemotherapy: around 70 percent of children who need chemotherapy to fight certain cancers end up with hearing loss.[19] Some of the most effective cancer-fighting medications have the unfortunate side effect of severely damaging the cochlea. A drug that saves the cochlea could easily reduce the effectiveness of the chemotherapy to cure the cancer. Finding a drug that is well tolerated, effective at rescuing hearing, and doesn't interfere with the effectiveness of other drugs is possible . . . it takes a lot of trial and error through experiments, and these experiments have to be done carefully to protect the health and well-being of those participating in the research. That's why we aren't there yet.

What about stem cells? These seem to be reported by the popular news media as the Fountain of Youth! It's true, stem cells carry some real promise. They can be coaxed into turning into lots of different cells in the body—cells that don't naturally regenerate in people, like nerve cells or sensory cells in the cochlea.[20] But how do you get them to go into the right spot, and connect with the nerves and other cells around them in a way that helps? Can it be done surgically, without doing more damage to the area you're trying to repair? If you do get stem cells in the right place, and they make good connections with nerves and other cells around, how do you make them grow just enough to help, but not keep growing and turning into a tumor? That could actually happen: stem cells multiply and take hold where they are supposed to, but don't know when to "turn off" and so grow into a tumor.[21]

I posed a lot of these questions to hearing researchers who study these kinds of problems, and here's what I've come to understand: it is likely that some drugs will be developed that will help rescue the hearing of people whose cochleas are injured by noise or some other trauma. These hearing-rescue drugs won't cure deafness, but they will lessen how much damage would have been done.[22] The damage might be lessened enough that instead of getting very little benefit from hearing aids, the hearing loss isn't so great and hearing aids are beneficial and they don't have to go so far as to get a CI. Eventually, stem cell researchers will likely find a way to implant stem cells and regrow the delicate sensory cells in ears that were injured (say, by premature birth or a side effect of medications), to the point where they don't need a CI and can use hearing aids instead.[23] Or, perhaps stem cells can help improve hearing nerve function, and make a CI more effective. It is not as likely that stem cells can help children whose genes didn't code for forming the delicate sensory cells in the first place. But, it is still quite possible that gene therapy plus stem cells can give children born deaf some hearing, so that they could benefit from hearing aids, or hybrid CI-hearing aid devices.

SHOULD A PARENT OF A CHILD WITH SEVERE-TO-PROFOUND HEARING LOSS HOLD OFF ON GETTING CIS TO SEE IF GENE THERAPY OR STEM CELL RESEARCH WILL CURE THE DEAFNESS?

This question has been posed a number of times in my fifteen years as a pediatric audiologist. When a CI electrode array is inserted in the cochlea, it typically wipes out any leftover scrap of hearing that was in the cochlea. What if gene therapy or stem cells could coax the ear into repairing itself, but only in an ear that never got a CI? There's a pretty straightforward answer: if the brain is going to make use of sound (ever) it needs to be stimulated with sound as soon as possible (via hearing aids or CIs). The brain doesn't stay perfectly accepting of new sound years down the road. Currently, the FDA approves CI in children aged twelve months and older. If CI is the best way to give clear access to sound, the sooner the brain gets the stimulation, the better. Babies implanted at age twelve months (and have good parental support, strong innate communication drive, etc.) typically catch up in speech and language to their normal-hearing peers by kindergarten. The outcome is less certain when children don't have much in the way of auditory stimulation the first few years of life, then all of a sudden get a CI. In fact, research has suggested that if hearing hasn't been a part of a child's life for the first seven years, the sound provided by a CI (given at age seven years or older) is not so easily used by the brain.[24] The brain may not be all that effective at decoding the sound from the CI, even after a lot of therapy. If hearing is to be a significant part of a child's experience, it isn't a good idea to hold off on CIs (or hearing aids) just in case a breakthrough in stem cell research comes along. At present, it's all about getting good language (ASL or spoken) into children's brains by whatever means makes sense for the family. At present, if spoken language is a goal, devices are part of the path.

6

BEYOND DEVICES: HOW DO YOU KNOW INTERVENTIONS ARE WORKING?

The whole point of hearing screenings, hearing tests, fitting devices, and putting time and effort into therapy sessions is to give the child with hearing loss access to language. And there's a *lot* more to intervention than simply fitting devices to a child to help that child hear better. So, how do we know if the plan is working? The development of language is a slow process, which means it can be hard to tell if progress is being made. The uncertainty whether interventions are effective can be deeply concerning, leaving families in a state of constant vigilance, or exhaustion, or both. This chapter looks at how to tell if the efforts of parents, teachers, therapists, and healthcare providers are actually helping.

WHAT IS "NORMAL" CHILDHOOD DEVELOPMENT?

"Normal" is a little bit of a gray area: it's what most of the rest of (healthy) babies of a certain age are able to do. Babies' brains and bodies continuously build new skills with every passing moment and experience. And it's through their experiences that they make developmental gains, one skill building upon another.[1] Let's take, for example, development of "gross motor" abilities in a baby. A newborn has limited ability to maneuver herself in her environment. Mostly, she can kick her legs, arch her back, roll her head side to side, move her arms, suck and swallow, and cry. Sometimes, a newborn baby will bring her fist to her mouth, and suck on her fist. A lot of the moving around is reflexive. That is, a newborn will wave his arms around with hands open and fingers out if not swaddled, as though he is trying to figure out where he is and why he's not being snuggled. But his waving of his hands is not intentional. If he's hungry, he cries. There's no forethought or planning, or expectation. There's just, "This is how I feel right now, so this is how I'm going to behave." As the newborn gets older, say, between ages one to three months, he starts doing new things, like lifting his head up when you have him do "tummy time." Being able to lift his head takes a lot of muscle training and learning how to control his big head, and starts with being able to move it from side to side as a newborn. Being able to lift his head, after all the strength training and practice controlling his head, means he has achieved a "developmental milestone." People who work with children pay lots of attention when children are meeting their developmental milestones, and if these milestones are achieved at appropriate ages. These "checkpoints" of development are a window into the bigger picture of what's going on with the child, day to day, in building new skills.

Babies develop their skills at different paces: some babies make fast progress socially (making great eye contact, smiling, laughing, etc.) but are slow to learn how to sit up on their own. Sometimes the opposite happens: quick to develop gross motor skills, but not so fast to mature socially. To continue the example of gross motor development, a baby is expected to roll from her stomach onto her back (without help from a parent) between ages four and seven months. If a baby isn't rolling over by seven months, this raises concern about the lag in meeting this gross motor milestone. Generally speaking, a baby wouldn't learn to crawl if he isn't able to roll from his back onto his stomach, and push up onto all-fours. If he isn't able to crawl, he probably won't build enough leg, arm, and body strength to be able to pull himself up to stand while holding onto furniture. If he doesn't pull up to stand, he won't build the leg and body strength to take his first steps . . . and so on. In our example here, it starts with rolling from back onto belly.

With language, babies with normal hearing are being bathed in spoken language daily. This "bathing in spoken language" is like constant tummy-time for the auditory and language centers of the brain: every experience is training the brain what to do with this complicated thing we call language. A baby aged one to three months old with normal hearing, and who is able to turn his head side-to-side while lying on his back, might alert to the sound of a parent's voice and orient his head to look toward the voice. This is early sound localization! Young babies also (generally) startle to loud sounds, and are awakened during nap if someone makes a noise that's too loud (much to the sleep-deprived parents' frustration). Young babies make cooing noises, as well as gurgles and cries. A baby can feel the tickle of her vocal cords vibrating, and might play with how this feels differently when she has her mouth open versus having her mouth closed when making noise. Depending on their hearing status, babies also hear these sounds that they are making. When a baby hears himself make these sounds, he is learning a sense of control over himself and how he interacts with the world around him, using his voice. As babies get older, maybe between six and twelve months, some delight in making an incredibly shrill screeching noise, over and over again. They may even laugh when they see people around them react by wincing and covering their ears. And then shriek again to see if they can make their parents wince again.

As babies start being able to sit up (between about five and seven months, or so) they start having little babbling "conversations" where they string together sounds, like "babababa." A baby might change the pitch of her voice up and down. All this vocal sound-play is evidence the baby is getting enjoyment from making these noises, either because she thinks it's cool to hear these sounds that she's making, or because it feels good in her throat and chest, or both. Babies with normal hearing, and many babies with hearing loss, babble like this. Sometimes, parents of children with hearing loss are able to recall subtle differences in how their child with hearing loss babbled compared to a sibling with normal hearing. But parents could drive themselves crazy trying to be master babbling-detectives, comparing any two children. Children develop differently anyway, so it's not worth making yourself go crazy (there's enough other stuff about parenting that will drive you crazy naturally, without going to look for it).

As parents, we engage with our babies as they babble, imitating their babbling sounds, and end up having little turn-taking "conversations" with them. This is highly rewarding for both the baby and the parents! Imagine, the baby babbles "amamama" and then pauses, and her mother says "Mamama?" and the baby babbles back to her mother "amamaMA!" And then her mother laughs. The baby smiles and claps her hands, so *very* proud of herself for making these noises! This kind of turn-taking babbling play is an early building block of verbal communication. We take turns when we talk with one another. It is part of our rules of communication, and babies learn these rules through this kind of babbling play with a "communication" partner. If a baby has hearing loss and isn't accessing spoken language through devices, his babbling often ends up being more one-sided. He may attend to your face, and if you are close he may hear you (especially if his hearing loss is a mild to moderate degree). But it might be harder to engage with him in the turn-taking game, because it might not be obvious to him when you are making vocal sounds, and when you are pausing. You might still be making babbling noises at him, but if he doesn't hear your babbling noises, he might think you've paused and he starts his turn, prematurely.

Babies who are making good strides in meeting their developmental milestones in language go from simple babbling, with only a few consonant sounds (like "b, d, m,") followed by the same vowel sound ("bababa" or "dadada"), to more sophisticated babbling: for example, "mamada-igdee." Babies with hearing loss who aren't accessing spoken language through devices don't often move from simple babbling into the more sophisticated babbling, at least, not without help (but we'll get to that shortly). This more sophisticated babbling usually happens for babies with normal hearing around age eight to ten months, and is a precursor to the baby's first "real" word. By "real" word we mean a symbol that carries with it a specific meaning, and is used on purpose. As the child nearing her first birthday continues to figure out how to make new sounds and new consonant-vowel combinations, she's been watching and listening to her caretakers (her language role-models) as they make lots of really complicated sounds quickly back and forth with their mouths (she's eavesdropping on your conversations). Eavesdropping is imperative to normal spoken language acquisition. Her first words are, in large part, motivated by her interest in moving from being an eavesdropper to an active participant in the conversation.

In normal day-to-day activities, parents describe what's happening in a silly, narrating-kind of game. Imagine trying to get a cheeky twelve-month-old to eat pureed vegetables, and he's pursing his lips together, not letting you shove the spoon in his mouth. He has a very clearly understood nonverbal gesture when you try to feed him: shaking his head "No!" . . . but you take a scoop of the vegetable pap, hold the spoon up high (making sure he sees the spoon), and you say "Joey, get ready! The airplane is coming in for a landing! Vrooom!!!" as you "fly" the spoon down to come in for a landing (and get the precious little angel to open his mouth and let you feed him). This little narrating game you just did with Joey to get him to take a bite of dinner was very rich in language stimulation. The "airplane" makes a noise: Vrooomm!! Maybe the "airplane" even makes some loops on its way to come in for a landing, and makes different noises as it makes loops. Use of these different sounds, combined with what's called "symbolic play" (the spoon becomes an imaginary airplane), brings additional meaning to the noises we make with our mouths, and is very motivating to get the child to participate, because it's play, and play is fun.

My oldest, Danielle (seven years old at the time of this writing), said her first intentional word when she was fourteen months old. It was in the bathtub, and we were playing with bath toys. She had taken a liking to a toy turtle. This turtle would dive into the soapy water, and come out, and dive in again, and sometimes even squirt water out of its mouth. One day in the bathtub, she said "tudle!" (her approximation for "turtle"). And she said it a couple more times that day in the tub, and not long after, a few more words started coming out of her: all words that were ones we had said over and over again to her, for at least the past several months, if not her whole life. I don't recall, but it's safe to say that when we gave Danielle a bath, we would describe what her different bath toys were doing as we played with them. I'm sure we also narrated what *she* did with them: "Oh, did the turtle fall off the boat?" we might say when she picked the turtle up from a floating toy boat and dropped it in the water. Hearing her parents say "turtle" hundreds of times during her first fourteen months was priming Danielle's developing auditory and language centers in her brain to make this word available to her as her first word. Nowadays, I can tell that when Danielle is old enough to have a cell phone, she better be on a plan with unlimited minutes . . . she's pretty chatty.

These above examples ("the airplane coming in for a landing" and the "turtle falling off the boat") are part of normal parent–child interactions. These interactions foster cognitive development as well as language acquisition. When a child engages in symbolic play (the spoon as an imaginary airplane), this shows the child has met a cognitive developmental milestone. Joey knows the spoon isn't an airplane, but he gets that this is a game and he goes with it. This is an example how language fosters cognitive development, and vice versa. One way to think about "cognition" and cognitive development is this is how a child's brain makes sense of his world, and how to navigate his way through it. As cognition develops, language becomes an integral part of this navigation through the world. If a child is hungry, sitting on the floor and crying isn't very helpful at getting his parent to understand what he wants. But if he gets out the word "Baba!" between cries, that makes it obvious what he wants. The cries are a nice additional motivator, using vocal sound, to get what he wants (and get it faster)!

Children usually say their first words between about twelve months and sixteen months. Again, children develop at different rates, with different skills acquired faster than others. A speech-language pathologist described to me that when a child is really learning how to get from one place to another faster (that is, learning she can run, not just cruise along furniture), she can get completely focused on her "motor." And this might leave little room for her to focus on developing language.[2] That said, toddlers should have at least a couple words that an unfamiliar adult can understand by the time they are eighteen months old. Some pediatricians take a more conservative approach, looking to see if a child will start saying some words between eighteen to twenty-two months before getting the child evaluated for possible speech-language delay. Others are more aggressive and recommend that children who are not expressing themselves verbally by the time they are eighteen months old be evaluated by a speech-language pathologist to see if there is a speech-language delay, and if speech-language therapy is indicated.

HOW DOES HEARING LOSS INFLUENCE "NORMAL" CHILD DEVELOPMENT?

Children with hearing loss are at risk for speech-language delay, as well as cognitive and social-emotional delays. In reality, these three areas of child development are highly interwoven, so it's not as though there are three separate, distinct aspects of child development that are at risk.[3] But, delays in one area impact the other two.

Having a hearing loss doesn't *guarantee* the child will have a speech-language delay, but the odds are pretty high that he or she will. As soon as a child is diagnosed with a permanent hearing loss, he should be enrolled in early intervention to begin receiving therapy from child-development specialists. What therapies and who provides them (and where) depends a lot on how old the child is, the extent of the delays, family wishes, and a myriad of other reasons. In a young baby, therapy services might first take on the form of "developmental play" to ensure the baby is making progress toward meeting his gross motor developmental milestones. Why gross motor, and not speech and language? It's easier for a baby to engage in turn-taking babbling "conversations" if he is able to sit up and hold his head up. First things first. Making sure these gross motor milestones are achieved on time helps set the stage for engaging in more directed speech and language therapy. Children diagnosed with hearing loss after the newborn period, who have shown good developmental progress in general, may have therapies that are focused exclusively on speech-language development, rather than on general development. Each child's situation is individual; the child, and his or her family ecosystem, are unlike anyone else's. When a child is referred to an early intervention (EI) provider, an evaluation of the child's strengths and challenges is to be completed within forty-five days of contact. The EI program drafts a report outlining the findings from the evaluation; describes whether or not the child qualifies for services, based on these findings; and if therapy is indicated, outlines which therapies and how often they should be provided. Then, with the family's input, the EI provider writes up an Individualized Family Service Plan (abbreviated IFSP). The IFSP is an agreement between the EI provider and the family that outlines what services the child and family will receive. These services can include speech and language therapy, developmental stimulation (which often takes on the form of "purposeful play"), physical therapy and/or occupational therapy (if indicated), and perhaps the services of other specialists. For instance, if the family wishes ASL to be incorporated into the child's language development services, provision of an ASL instructor may be included in the IFSP, where the ASL instructor comes to the family's house and teaches the *family* ASL. The family, of course, is the language role model for a child, and to be that role model, their language skills need to be ahead of the child's. So, teaching the family ASL is, in fact, providing (family-centered) interventions for the child. A brief note: in most states, simply having a permanent hearing loss (whether there's a delay in speech and language, or not) automatically entitles a child, aged zero to three years, to EI services. Find out for sure what your child is entitled to by asking your child's clinicians, EI service provider, and other parents. A couple organizations that can help you figure out what your child is entitled to: the Federation for Children with Special Needs (www.fcsn.org) and Parent to Parent USA (www.P2Pusa.org).

Quite often, the therapies provided to a child are incorporated into typical, routine activities you're already doing, but perhaps with some adjustments. For instance, when reading a book to a child, a developmental specialist might recommend that rather than turn the page after you finish reading the words on the page, spend more time on each page, really looking at and describing the pictures you see. In *The Three Little Pigs and the Big Bad Wolf,* can you point out the color of the straw that the first pig built his house out of? What clothes is that first little pig wearing? Are there trees in the picture (and how many)? If there are trees, is the color of the leaves the same color as the grass? Can you say "green" and, while keeping your child's joint visual attention, do the ASL sign for "green" to describe the color of the leaves in the trees and the grass? Does it sound like it will take a while to get through a book this way? Yes. But it's time much better spent stimulating language than reading quickly through ten different books and briefly glancing at the pictures.

As the developmental specialists work with the baby with hearing loss, part of this work is bringing caregivers into the activities, to show the parents the kinds of things they can do to support the child's progress. A very effective therapist helps the parents see themselves as the child's role model, and helps the parents identify a child's efforts that should be acknowledged and celebrated. This is another aspect of managing childhood hearing loss in a family-centered way.

When a child has a hearing loss, this puts limitations on that child's ability to eavesdrop on conversations. One way this limitation has been described is to consider that we all have a "listening bubble" and the size of that bubble depends on our hearing sensitivity. If our hearing is normal, we have a normal-sized listening bubble (easily the size of a kitchen or living room). A conversation happening inside that listening bubble is overheard. If a person has hearing loss, his or her listening bubble is smaller (compared to the person with normal hearing). A conversation that would have been inside a normal-sized listening bubble (that is, overheard) might fall outside the smaller listening bubble of someone with hearing loss (that is, not heard). Devices help to make a smaller-than-normal listening bubble bigger; but there's more to listening with this device-supplemented listening bubble than just turning them on and assuming all is normal. Parents should continue the usual narrating activities that they would do if their child had normal hearing. They should continue reading books to their child, and playing vocal games with him, blowing raspberries, and taking delight in being silly with him! And, as much as possible, narrate more often (think of the richer narration of *The Three Little Pigs* example above). It might feel a little foreign at first, but describe to your child everything you are doing. For instance, when you are cooking, instead of silently walking to a cupboard and pulling out a pot, filling with water and putting on the stove, say out loud, "Okay, now we're going to the cupboard and getting out the pot. We have to start boiling water, so we need to fill up the pot with water from the faucet . . ." and so on. Children need to hear words over and over, in the context of how these words are used, before they understand what they mean. The "pot with boiling water" will be a "pot that's getting washed with soap and water" after we are done cooking; that is, the words "pot" and "water" mean this big metal thing and this wet stuff, but these words are used differently in the two different contexts (cooking vs. cleaning). Firsthand knowledge of how "pot" and "water" are used in different ways helps a child generalize what these two words actually mean (that *specific* metal thing you cook with, and that wet stuff I can splash in and drink). When a child has hearing loss, it's hard to predict just how often he actually hears a word said in his vicinity. What if he heard really well when you described "boiling water in the pot" but he didn't hear so well that you were using "soap and water to wash the pot?" Stack the deck in his favor by describing your actions all the time. And as much as possible, do this with hearing aids/CIs on, as this expands his listening bubble so that it's easier for him to overhear your narration. Particularly when the activity requires listening, such as reading a book, it's important to have the child's hearing aids/CIs on. Rough-housing on the living room floor, giving piggy-back rides, and tickling: it's not as important that the hearing aids or CIs be on. All things being equal, hearing aids/CIs should be on during all "awake" hours and nonwater (e.g., bath time) activities. But, if the child pulls the hearing aids out in the middle of running around in the back yard with a parent or sibling, it might make sense to just let him run, and not stop everything to make him put hearing aids back in. That could feel like a punishment . . . and it's important to keep the use of hearing aids/CIs something the child is praised for using, and not punished for taking out. Watching movies or cartoons? Hearing aids should be in so she can hear the characters. It's safe to make it an expectation that hearing aids must be in to watch television. At dinner time, families might make rules, such as "No cell phones at the dinner table, and hearing aids are on." But pick and choose when listening is most important in a child's day, and prioritize when hearing aids or CIs must be used, and when it's okay to take a break from them.

In all of these usual daily routines, can you tell if the hearing aids or CIs help your child to hear better? Does your child pay attention longer to a book you're reading when he's using his hearing aids? Does he like a cartoon more when his hearing aids are in? Does he get really close to the television when he doesn't have his hearing aids in, and doesn't go so close when he *does* have them in? Does he make more sounds with his voice when his hearing aids are in? Or less sounds when his hearing aids are in? Or, does it seem like his behavior and attention are the same, whether his hearing aids are in or not?

In chapter 5, I briefly mentioned babies and toddlers take their hearing aids out, and it can become a battle of wills to get them to use the hearing aid. Sometimes it's just a phase, but sometimes the child is trying to tell you something: "Take this thing out. It's not doing anything." If the child is rejecting her hearing aids, this behavior is communicating *something*. Maybe it's her way of expressing her independence (a phase), or maybe she knows something you and the audiologist need to know ("something's wrong with my device"). On the flip side, I've had parents tell me at appointments that their early-rising toddler comes into their room every morning and brings them her hearing aids, as if to say, "You need to put these in so I can start my day!" If children figure out they are getting benefit from their hearing aids, they tend to accept them (notwithstanding those challenging behavioral phases). And some of the best ways to help a child figure out she is benefiting from her hearing aids is to experience listening activities with her, while she's using her hearing aids. Reading books, playing with sound-making toys (especially sound makers that also light up when the sound is activated), and playing a musical instrument are all great listening activities. Music exposure from a young age is an amazing way to enrich a child's brain, whether he or she has hearing loss or not. And the type of music doesn't matter; although live music, rather than recorded, means the child can see someone in the room is actively making this sound. It's not just pressing the "play" button on the stereo, it's sitting down at the piano or guitar, and reading music to know what to play. And what's even better about live music? When it's not played perfectly every time, like it is in a recorded song. Catching a mistake in a note that was played shows excellent auditory awareness. The mistakes a musician makes when playing a song might be a bit subtle, but if you know the song, you can tell if the wrong note was played at the wrong time. The timing might be right (that is, the rhythm), but the pitch of the note played is wrong. This kind of sound awareness, of picking up on the wrong note played, is good for all children. And it can be as simple as playing "Mary Had a Little Lamb" on a toy xylophone, to as grandiose as playing Bach on a baby grand piano. Of course, singing is the easiest music stimulation: sing often! Even if you can't carry a tune to save your life. If you sing or play music for auditory stimulation, I urge you to purposely play the wrong note, stop everything, make a face toward the child, laugh, and say "No! No! That isn't right!" and play it wrong again! Stop, make the grimacing face again, and say "That wasn't right either!" and then play it correctly, and then stop and cheer yourself. What does your child do? Clap because you played it right? Want you to play it wrong over and over? Whatever you do, this kind of musical play is golden. For children with normal hearing, and hearing loss.

So far, we've briefly covered some general topics around child development, and only briefly touched on the influence of hearing loss on normal childhood development. It is my own personal opinion that if a parent should focus efforts on any particular topic, it's on learning how kids develop at a normal pace, and working with child-development specialists to identify your child's individual strengths to foster his or her development in all areas. And every child has individual strengths. Those innate strengths are a foundation for a child at risk for delays to progress right along at a normal rate.

Management of childhood hearing loss is about breaking down the barriers to normal development as effectively as possible, so that hearing loss is only a characteristic of your child, and not the single thing that defines him. There's a lot more child in there than a "deaf kid." You may notice that much of the way I phrase things in this book is "a child with hearing loss" rather than "hearing-impaired child." Because, in my opinion, the child comes first, and the hearing loss is secondary. What about your child's personality? What are his quirks? Is he serious? Silly? How does he behave differently around different adults and different children? Who does he seem to like better? All these "nonhearing" aspects of your child are what defines his identity, not his hearing loss. That's a factor to contend with, for sure, but only as a barrier to you getting to know him. So how do we do this?

VERIFICATION AND VALIDATION OF DEVICES TO ASSIST WITH HEARING

From the perspective of a clinician, whether or not an intervention works defines if we are doing our job well. Figuring out if an intervention is working takes on two forms: verification, and validation. These words seem pretty similar, and in general conversation, they are. From a clinical perspective, they are markedly different. The word "verification" means something quite different from "validation" in a clinical sense. Recall in chapter 5, I mentioned that the only way to know if hearing aids are working is if the audiologist uses special equipment, including a thin flexible tube and microphone, to tell how much sound the hearing aid is sending into the child's ear canal. This test is called "real-ear measures" (and is also referred to as "probe-microphone measures" and "real ear verification"). And it is just that: it is a verification that the hearing aids are working as they are intended to. These sophisticated little mini-computer-hearing aids programmed by the audiologist according to a prescription for how much sound is appropriate, based on the hearing test results. But how do we really know if the *predicted* output of the hearing aid is what actually happens in the ear? The only way to know this is with real-ear/probe-microphone measures. The results of this test tell the audiologist what speech sounds fall into the child's residual auditory area, and if any sounds are boosted too loud. This test also shows what sounds aren't boosted enough to be heard by the child. It guides the audiologist in figuring out if these inaudible sounds (too quiet) can be boosted any further without causing louder sounds to be boosted too much. For children with severe (or greater) hearing loss, it can be extremely helpful in setting expectations regarding what they can, and cannot hear, with their hearing aids. It's certain they won't hear many of the soft sounds of speech, because they simply don't have enough residual auditory area to boost soft sounds without making the loud sounds too loud (or the hearing aids simply can't amplify the sound any further).

Another approach to verification of hearing aids is to test how well your child hears the audiologist's voice when he or she is in the test booth. There are special speech-tests where children are asked to repeat words the audiologist says, or point to pictures or objects (the audiologist says "point to the hotdog": does the child point to the picture of the hotdog, or to a picture of the airplane?).[4] These speech-understanding tests can be done with the child's hearing aids off, and with hearing aids on. Does the child do better with the hearing aids on? Whether or not these speech understanding tests can be done depends on whether or not the child has made good progress in learning language: if the test is simply "too old" for her, she'll do poorly whether her hearing aids are in or not, simply because she doesn't know the difference between (for instance) the word "hotdog" and the word "airplane."

Diagnostic hearing tests typically focus on figuring out where a child's hearing thresholds are: how soft a sound can the child hear?[5] But we don't listen to soft beeps when we talk with each other. So hearing aids aren't programmed to make soft beeps more audible: they are programmed to make speech more understandable. Testing a child's hearing in a sound booth using beeps, with his hearing aids on, is not a good way to figure out how well the hearing aids are working. The beeps used in hearing testing are not anything like speech, and hearing aids with current technology "know" this. They don't boost these beeps very much, most of the time. So "aided audiograms" aren't used much anymore as a way to verify if hearing aids are working. Speech understanding testing and probe-microphone measures are much more useful.

The opposite is true with CIs and bone-conduction hearing systems. When these devices are programmed, they are often verified by testing a child in the sound booth. These devices also cannot be verified using probe-microphones. Children with adequate sound from their CIs or bone-conduction hearing systems have "aided" hearing thresholds that are in, or close to, the normal hearing range. Speech-understanding tests can also be done to help verify that the devices are actually helping. When to use these kinds of speech tests depends on how much spoken language the child has acquired.

Do these verification tests jive with a parent's observations? They should. If they don't, it's worth spending some time figuring out why. If the hearing aids are putting out great sound, and *should* be giving good stimulation, but the parents report the child doesn't respond to much sound at all whether hearing aids are in or out, why is that? Sometimes bringing in the child development/EI specialist to the audiologist appointment is helpful when this situation arises. Often, the audiologist will simply ask for parents' observations about what their child does, or doesn't do, while using her devices. Some of the most common answers are related to awareness of environmental sound (door closing, dog barking, car horn honking, etc.) and awareness of voices. Of course, a great way to tell if devices are helping is if the child is learning to use new words to express himself.

Thankfully, there are excellent questionnaires that have been developed to help tease out whether or not a child is doing better with devices, or if the devices aren't helping very much. The Early Listening Function (ELF) for infants and toddlers[6] and Children's Home Inventory of Listening Difficulties (CHILD)[7] are excellent tools that parents can use at home to get a better sense of what their child can, and cannot hear, with and without devices on. The ELF is a questionnaire developed by audiologist Karen Anderson, PhD, and is appropriate for children aged newborn to three years old. The ELF is very user-friendly, and gives the parents a chance to uncover specifics about what their child can hear, and what he or she can't. This can be very empowering for parents, particularly for very young children. The CHILD is a tool developed by audiologist Joseph Smaldino, PhD, and is appropriate for children aged three to twelve years. The CHILD specifically looks at how well the child communicates in the family environment, and can help identify when remote microphone technology (like an FM system) might be a good idea to start using. Ultimately, it's the parents' opinion that matters most regarding whether or not the devices are giving the child what he or she needs. These questionnaires truly tap into "validation" of management efforts, which is a far higher bar to achieve than simply testing hearing, or even verifying the function of the devices.

EARLY INTERVENTION AND SCHOOL-BASED SERVICES

Early intervention services are provided for children age zero to three years. Once children turn three, they become eligible for services from the special-education program in your local public school system. Yes: two years before most kids go to kindergarten, a child with special developmental needs (such as having hearing loss) is eligible to receive services from the public school system. And the school system receives federal funding to assist in meeting the needs of children with developmental and educational challenges. The basis for the public school systems to be tasked with meeting the needs of children with developmental needs is the Individuals with Disabilities Education Act (abbreviated

IDEA).[8] This is an educational Bill of Rights for children with developmental challenges that would impact their ability to receive a free, appropriate, public education. That is, in the United States, it is considered a constitutional right (and society's obligation) for every child to be granted an education. And this includes children with disabilities. For those of you who want to dig more deeply into understanding educational rights, there is a rich history, going back to the Rehabilitation Act of 1973 and has since involved several laws and court cases. In summary, access to an appropriate education is a civil right, protected by the Equal Protection Clause of the Fourteenth Amendment of the US Constitution. And, just because one child needs more help to do well does not mean that child's family has to "foot the bill." Disability can happen in anyone's family, and so it is every family's responsibility to pool our resources so that all children can go to school and have a chance at a good education. A short, although fairly dense, one-page overview of the IDEA can be found at http://www.apa.org/about/gr/issues/disability/idea.aspx.[9] There is also a ton of information about IDEA, services for zero to three years ("Part C"—early intervention services) and services for three to twenty-one years ("Part B"—special education and related services) at http://idea.ed.gov/.

When a child with hearing loss is nearing his third birthday, if he has been receiving services through an EI provider, there should be a transition to receiving services through the public school. A phone call to the school's special-education department can initiate that process, and typically involves the EI provider (zero to three years) assisting in the transition to the special-education department (three to twenty-one years). There is an evaluation process for the school personnel to understand what are the child's specific educational needs. After this evaluation, the school drafts and Individualized Education Plan (abbreviated IEP). This plan is an agreement between the family and school that describes the kind of services the child will receive, including who will provide the services, how often they will be provided, and what the goals are. This plan is reviewed in a meeting between the parents and special-education administrators and personnel. Most often, reports from the child's healthcare providers play a part in helping to clarify what a child's educational needs are, in light of his or her disability. Specific to our topic: an audiologist's, speech-language pathologist's, and ENT physician's reports might all be part of the clinical documentation that clarifies the need for educational support services. These services might include speech-language therapy, extra tutoring, reading assistance, resource room time, extra time for taking tests, and communication of assignments in writing sent home to parents. Also, it is *very* common for an FM system to be recommended (particularly, recommended by the audiologist) to assist the child with hearing loss hear the teacher better. As noted in previous chapters, school classrooms are usually difficult listening environments, even for a child with normal hearing. Before a child is in a structured classroom, teacher-to-child interaction is very often one on one or in small groups. In a setting like that, a child with hearing loss typically is engaged directly by the teacher/parent/daycare provider. When the number of students per teacher (that is, the "student to teacher ratio") gets pretty big, the teacher can't engage with any particular student more than the others on a routine basis and still be a good teacher for the whole class. For instance, in a daycare with two teachers and eight kids, that's a four-to-one ratio of child to teacher. In a typical first-grade classroom, there might be twenty-five children with one teacher (and maybe a teacher's assistant/teacher's aide).

Technology that piggy-backs on the hearing aids/CIs (that is, an FM system) can easily bring the teacher's voice right to that student who truly needs to hear clearly and consistently. In chapter 5, I noted that children who use devices really need to use an FM system in school, because the distance between teacher and student has a huge impact on how well the teacher is heard. There are several different kinds of FM systems available, so which one is the right one? It is most appropriate for the audiologist to specify the system that would work best for the individual student. All things being equal, an FM system that connects directly with the hearing aids or CIs sounds best. However, there may be reasons this creates a challenge for the student, so each child's circumstances should be considered on an individual basis. Some school systems have the luxury of having an "educational audiologist" on staff or available as a consultant. Those audiologists who are specifically trained in working with students with hearing loss in their classroom are an exceptional resource to both school and family. Audiologists with this particular knowledge base are typically the most current in their knowledge of available FM technology, the pros and cons of different systems for a particular student, and can best advise the IEP process. If your school district does not have an educational audiologist on staff or available as a consultant, include this as a request in your child's IEP, particularly if there have been issues with the FM system being used consistently.

When the FM system is provided as part of an educational support listed in the IEP, it is the school's responsibility to make sure the system is working well (and this includes having the system checked at least annually for maintenance) and that teachers know how to use and care for the system. Teacher in-service training by an audiologist on the correct use and care of the FM system should be written into the IEP, and not be assumed this is understood. While everyone may have good intentions to do right by the student with hearing loss, if the FM system isn't working from Day 1, the child might not know what he or she is missing! Knowing how to use the system, troubleshoot problems, and what to do if the system breaks is the teacher's responsibility (and the school's responsibility to the teacher). FM systems are generally fairly easy to use, so long as they are set up correctly and the teachers are shown how to tell if it's working, and what to do if it's not. FM system "cheat sheets" can really come in handy: things like "make sure the microphone cord is plugged into the system" and details about how to tell if the FM system is charged up, or the battery is dead. Some good general information about FM systems is available at http://www.betterhearing.org/hearing-loss-children/classroom.[10] Since technology changes pretty quickly, a search on manufacturers' websites might give you the most up-to-date information about FM systems: on the website for Phonak www.phonak.com[11] (a manufacturer of many devices to assist people with hearing loss), in the Search box on the home page, typing in "Pediatric Solutions FM" brings up some good parent- and teacher-directed materials. On the website for Oticon www.oticon.com [12] (another manufacturer of devices to assist people with hearing loss), in the Search box on the home page, typing in "FM system" brings up a number of links to information about FM systems that are appropriate for parents and teachers. On both websites, though, these searches also bring up technical reports and audiologist-directed materials. If the information looks denser than is helpful, check out another link! And, of course, ask your child's audiologist to provide you and the teacher with materials that are helpful about FM systems.

THE SIFTER

So do the hearing aids/CIs and FM system work in helping a particular child hear better in the classroom? Tests can be run to verify if the hearing aids, CIs, and even the FM system are working well, but that doesn't mean the child is performing well, academically. Just as parent observations are so important in validating the audiological management plan in general, teacher observations are vital in validating the audiological management plan outside of home. How well does the student follow spoken instruction? How often does the child participate in class, such as raising his or her hand to answer a question posed by the teacher? How well does the child get along with other kids in school?

Although childhood hearing loss is considered fairly common compared to other childhood conditions that could warrant the need for educational supports, a teacher in a mainstream public school setting may have only a handful of students with hearing loss during his or her career. There may be several years between having a student with hearing loss in class. While teachers are expert in educating their class, they may not have considerable experience with the specific educational needs of a student with hearing loss. In the same vein, a parent is the expert at raising his or her child with hearing loss, but is not necessarily an expert on hearing loss. The IEP is intended to support the teacher, as well as the student, in achieving the educational goals for that child. But, the IEP process is flexible by design, and the IEP should be modified if the plan isn't meeting the student's or teacher's needs. If a particular student is having difficulties in the classroom, how do we know if it is due to his hearing loss versus waning motivation to do well in school in general? The hearing loss shouldn't be a crutch, or the go-to excuse for poor academic performance. Fortunately, there is an excellent, carefully designed questionnaire for teachers to screen for educational difficulties in students who have hearing loss: the Screening Instrument for Targeting Educational Risk (SIFTER).[13] It turns out, the SIFTER is also pretty good at picking up on children who are only *suspected* of having hearing loss (and should have their hearing checked to rule out hearing loss as an issue contributing to academic difficulties). The SIFTER was developed by Karen Anderson, PhD (I mentioned before, Dr. Anderson also developed the ELF questionnaire), and can be accessed at https://successforkidswithhearingloss.com/uploads/SIFTER.pdf (the manual for scoring and interpreting the SIFTER can be accessed at https://successforkidswithhearingloss.com/uploads/SIFTER_Manual.pdf). If the teacher has concerns that the student isn't doing very well in class, then this fifteen-item questionnaire can be helpful in figuring out "what do we do next?" If the teacher's answers to the SIFTER questions flag any particular issue, then further educational review and perhaps educational assessments are warranted. Sometimes, moving from one grade to the next shows certain vulnerabilities in the student's ability to manage his hearing loss, but these aren't immediately obvious as hearing-related. Is the student exhausted at the end of the school day, when he wasn't before? Is he struggling with math now, when he did very well in that subject the previous school year? It may be that both student and teacher are working very hard to succeed, but something about the material, or the way the student needs it to be taught, is creating a barrier. In such situations, a consulting Teacher of the Deaf and Hard-of-Hearing can review the material and methods of instruction, and recommend alternatives that might help the student more easily learn the challenging material. A Teacher of the Deaf and Hard-of-Hearing (often abbreviated TOD) is a teacher who has additional training and skills in teaching children with hearing loss. Teacher in-service training by a TOD is quite common, and is an educational support that would be written into the IEP.

What are the goals of the management plan for a child with hearing loss? It depends on who's asking. Is the goal to have a well-educated young adult graduate from high school, headed to college, reading at or above grade-level? Lots of parents would probably see that as an excellent goal. Is the goal to have a socially astute, happy young adult with lots of friends? That might be the highest priority for the student herself. Is the goal to keep the child in a mainstream public school classroom with normal-hearing peers, rather than have to attend a school program that is out-of-district and geared toward educating children with hearing loss? That might be on the minds of school administrators. Perhaps a goal is for the student to become a high-earning taxpayer. That might be a motivator for an elected representative who helps keep IDEA funding coming to a school district to support the special-education department. All of these goals can easily overlap, but they are sometimes in conflict. Children with excellent social skills tend to do better in the classroom than children who are socially challenged. Having fun and being popular at the expense of academics is a balancing act for any student and family. Being able to continue attending a mainstream public school program (rather than attend a school for the Deaf and Hard-of-Hearing) often means the child can attend school closer to home, and it costs the school system a lot less to educate him. But if the child needs that level of support, and the school is having budget shortfalls, there may be a real battle between the family and the school district. And, of course, it is in everyone's best interest for the child to succeed in fulfilling his potential, and be able to pursue career choices based on his innate potential and interests, rather than have his career choices limited by his hearing loss. However, in the United States, everyone has a say in how their tax dollars are spent, and generous educational funding might be less popular than cutting taxes in an election year. Many professionals (accountants, computer programmers, teachers, physicians, attorneys, and audiologists) were born with permanent hearing loss. Those successful people who have hearing loss certainly should be commended for the outrageous amount of effort it took to overcome the difficulties stemming from their hearing loss. Their families should be equally commended. But so should the school system and community that created the opportunities for students with hearing loss to meet their potential. In the end, no one wants efforts or resources to be wasted, and it's in everyone's best interest for the child to succeed. The best way for this to happen is for parents to be strong advocates for their child's needs, right from the start, but keep open communication with EI providers and school administrators, and keep the focus on the child's best interests. When parents, clinicians, and educators all see themselves on the same team, the interventions for childhood hearing loss can work pretty well.

7

MEMBERS OF THE MANAGEMENT TEAM

There is a laundry list of people who may be involved in helping to manage childhood hearing loss. Permanent childhood hearing loss is a condition that is well suited for a team approach for managing, rather than a single clinician-to-patient relationship, which is what most of us are familiar with when we get sick and see our primary care doctor. The needs of a child with hearing loss are varied, and no one professional has the breadth of knowledge and skills necessary to meet all these needs. But, it can be confusing which team member is responsible for what! There is often a lot of overlap in responsibilities, too, and sometimes there can be conflicting recommendations given to parents by members on the same team. What's a parent to do?

THE NECESSITY OF A TEAM APPROACH

Historically, most medical care was "siloed:" one clinician (most often a primary care doctor) was expert at taking care of a patient's medical problem, and either the patient got better, or he didn't, and the primary care doctor referred the patient to a specialist. Then, the care for that medical problem was mostly between the specialist and patient, with the primary care doctor kept informed but otherwise not directly involved in the medical care. This model of care taking place without much interaction between a primary clinician and additional participating healthcare providers works well when the medical problem is straightforward. A child with a sinus infection is miserable, but can usually be treated by the pediatrician who examines the sinuses and prescribes antibiotics to clear the infection. The child doesn't need to see a respiratory therapist to learn how to breathe through her mouth until her nose unclogs. Alternatively, a high-school athlete who tears a ligament in the knee may need care from an orthopedic surgeon, a physical therapist, and athletic trainer. These three members of the child's team have complementary roles: the surgeon provides the surgical repair of the damaged ligament, the physical therapist directs the recovery process, and the athletic trainer helps bring the athlete back into readiness for participating on the field again as well as monitor the athlete for signs of problems with that knee going forward. The orthopedic surgeon plays a role in clearing the athlete for participation in sports after recovery, and the physical therapist might provide the athletic trainer with a tailored strengthening plan to assist with future injury prevention.

The management of permanent childhood hearing loss requires teamwork, particularly early in the diagnostic and intervention process. Who is on the team depends in large part on the child's needs and the family's wishes, but in most every case, there will at least be an audiologist, otolaryngologist (ENT physician), speech-language pathologist, and pediatrician. And, of course, the child and parents/caregivers are integral members of this team. Why so many people for something as fundamental as hearing?

We have already established that hearing is a doorway for spoken language to get to the brain: if that doorway is closed off, there isn't as much language getting to the brain. So, this requires detailed understanding of the type and degree of hearing loss as well as ways to make that "doorway" open wider (these are in the audiologist's purview) as well as helping the brain figure out what to do with the sound and use it to acquire spoken language (this shifts into the speech-language pathologist's role, as well as some other providers). When permanent hearing loss is present in children, it might mean there is an underlying medical condition that needs to be detected and treated (part of the ENT physician's role). If parents want to identify if the cause of the hearing loss is genetic then, while there is not currently a treatment, it is in the ENT physician's scope to discuss with the family the benefits and risks of exploring genetic testing, and help to interpret the results in a way that empowers the family. For instance, finding out the cause of a child's hearing loss is due to genetics may influence how many more children the parents wish to have. Finding out that the hearing loss is genetic will mean the child with hearing loss will have a good idea what is the likelihood he himself will have children with hearing loss. Interpreting the results of genetic testing can get complicated, and what to do with this knowledge could be even more so. Sometimes a genetic counselor is brought in to help the parents understand the implications of test results. A genetic counselor is a professional with at least a master's degree in genetic counseling, and has been credentialed (either with state license or other credential) to provide clinical care.

Among many other responsibilities, the role of the speech-language pathologist might be first to figure out if there is a delay in speech or language, and if so, the extent of the delay. Sometimes the extent of the delay is described in "how many months behind" the child is. For instance, an eighteen-month-old who is making sophisticated babbling sounds, but not yet using any words, might be considered to be at a twelve-month equivalent age for *expressive* language (that is, using words or signs to get her message out). Since she's eighteen months old, this is equivalent to a six-month delay. This clinical examination of strengths versus delays is not intended to be a report card: rather, it helps to define how intensive therapy should be and where the challenges are most significant. Recall the review of developmental milestones in chapter 6. Documenting where a child is in meeting these checkpoints along the road to developing all the necessary skills for communication gives the speech-language pathologist the evidence needed to formulate the IFSP with the family (Individualized Family

Service Plan—the "alphabet soup" of terms for therapy, education, audiology and ENT is a language on its own).

As mentioned in the last chapter, when a child with hearing loss is enrolled in EI (birth to three years old), she is usually seen by a few different therapists. Who sees the child and when depends on the goals outlined in the IFSP. One therapist that will likely be part of the team is a developmental specialist. Often, these professionals have a background in early childhood education, with a particular focus on the development of children with special healthcare needs. They may engage the child in developmental play, which can be thought of as a general approach to motivating the child to make good progress in all areas of development: gross motor, fine motor, cognition, communication, and the like. As mentioned earlier in this book, gross motor development includes a baby being able to roll over from back to front, learning to crawl and walk, jump, and climb stairs. Fine motor development includes things like reaching out to grab a toy in front, picking up Cheerios and putting them in her mouth, and holding and scribbling with crayons. Cognitive development includes things like stranger anxiety and "object permanence" (putting a toy under a box on the floor doesn't mean the toy is gone forever . . . the toy still exists even though the baby can't see it, and so the baby tries to get it). And, of course, communication is about *receptive* language development (understanding what someone is communicating to the child) and expressive language development (the child getting his point across). Almost always, expressive language is a little (or a lot) further behind receptive language. When a well-meaning grandparent says "Oh, he understands everything you say, he's just not interested in saying anything yet," it rings with a little truth. Although, it's not necessarily about the child's interest: personally, I find this well-intentioned statement to sound a little judgmental. Why does expressive language lag receptive? Remember the story I conveyed about my oldest child, Danielle, saying "tudle" for the first time? She heard "turtle" in many different contexts (the turtle swimming, the turtle falling off the boat, the turtle squirting water out of its mouth) for months before "tudle" *clicked* in her head as the mental symbol for the word "turtle." Not only did she have to *know* what a turtle is, she had to have the coordination of her mouth, vocal cords, and breathing to make a word that was close enough to the correct word for her parents to understand! The developmental specialist identifies opportunities in the child's natural environment to help him practice his skills, and build them up to meet his developmental milestones.

Often, efforts to progress a child's ability to communicate verbally will be supplemented by introduction of simple signs (also known as "baby signs"), such as the signs for "more, eat, milk, up, all-done, and please." Baby sign is in vogue in many regions, and is often described as another way to engage with a child. The idea is that acquiring *any* language is good, and learning any symbol of meaning (that is, a word or a sign) will scaffold (that is, raise up) future language development. Often, developmental specialists will introduce signs and gestures to help a child in EI build a broader vocabulary for expressing his needs. This does not mean a decision is being made that the child will be taught ASL rather than being taught to speak. Those decisions are part of a discovery process and are the role of the parents, with input from members of the team.

If parents do want to explore ASL instruction to see how well their child makes progress using this mode of communication, it's best if this instruction is provided to the parents and any adult regularly involved with the child. And the ASL instructor needs to be someone who is actually fluent in ASL[1] (and it's a good idea to have this detail—that the ASL instructor is fluent—included in the IFSP). Ideally, the ASL instructor will also have cultural ties to the Deaf community, so that the family and child can have exposure to Deaf culture. This exposure should be offered in an unbiased way, with the ASL instructor sharing what he or she finds valuable about Deaf culture. EI professionals, like all people, carry biases and opinions formed by past experiences: biases can be acknowledged without attempting to sway parents in one direction or another.

When parents opt for their child with hearing loss to use hearing and spoken language as primary mode of communication, a certified Listening and Spoken Language Specialist (LSLS) is an important addition to the child's management team. This is particularly true when a child receives a CI, since the child needs to learn how to listen with it. An LSLS is perhaps the most qualified professional to work with a child who is a recent CI recipient. LSLS professionals are certified by the AG Bell Academy for Listening and Spoken Language, and typically have a background as a speech-language pathologist, Teacher of the Deaf and Hard-of-Hearing, or audiologist. The certification process to become an LSLS is quite extensive, and requires meeting eligibility requirements, passing a certifying exam, and completing continuing education. Often, this is in addition, and complementary to, maintaining professional licensure and skill set in one's background profession. As with inclusion of an ASL instructor, detailing the credentials of the LSLS in the IFSP is a good idea.[2] Given the LSLS's specialization in the optimal acquisition of spoken language in children who have hearing loss, it is clear they value the child being a member of the "hearing community." Parents should have an opportunity to learn about the LSLS's values, in a way that does not seek to sway the parents' decisions, or otherwise introduce bias. It is the parents' decision, with facts (not opinions) shared with the family to help make informed decisions related to their child's care.

EVOLVING NEEDS MEANS AN EVOLVING TEAM

As the child grows and matures, his management needs will change. There will be new members of the team who join, while others depart. When a child turns three years old, his team will probably include school-based special-education personnel. This will probably include a speech-language pathologist, and might include an educational audiologist. A Teacher of the Deaf and Hard-of-Hearing may also become a member of the team. Who joins at this time depends on the goals outlined in the IEP (Individualized Education Plan—there's that "alphabet soup" again), and who is necessary to help the child achieve those goals. Sometimes, there will be a need for short-term consultants to participate. For instance, the educational audiologist may identify the noise level in the classrooms are too high to allow the child with hearing loss to hear his teacher and peers, even with an FM system. In such cases, it is possible for the school to retain an acoustical engineer who can evaluate the classroom and recommend ways to retrofit the space to make it more hospitable to listening. In this event, the modifications to help the child with hearing loss benefit everyone else in the classroom too. Noisy classrooms make it hard for all students to learn, so damping down noisy heating and ventilation systems and other "building noise" helps everyone (including the teacher, who may have less vocal strain at the end of the day if she doesn't have to talk over the room noise).

On the medical side of things, the ENT physician and audiologist have complementary roles. As described in earlier chapters, the audiologist is often the entry point to hearing healthcare. This is particularly true if the child was referred for further testing after he or she didn't pass the newborn hearing screening. The initial identification of the presence of hearing loss is the role of the audiologist. When this happens, it is important to try to learn what caused the hearing loss: this is for the ENT physician to explore with the family. The audiologist may have specific test results that point to the root cause, and these are communicated to the ENT physician to factor into his or her clinical impression. The ENT physician has a number of tools available to figure out the cause, such as blood tests (including genetics testing), MRI and CT radiology tests, tests of how well other body organs are functioning (like the kidneys and heart), and tests for certain infections. On occasion, the cause of the hearing loss is associated with a medical problem, and the fact the hearing loss was identified meant the underlying medical problem was identified too. In fact, the hearing loss may have meant diagnosis of a medical problem much earlier than if hearing wasn't screened in the first place. For instance, there are certain (rare) conditions that affect the kidneys as well as hearing, and (even rarer) conditions that affect the heart and the ears. If such medical conditions are found, the ENT physician can coordinate treatment, and perhaps bring in other physicians to assist. And, of course, the ENT is tasked with the medical management of ear health issues, such as ear infections.

Pretty early on, the ENT physician will coordinate having the child's vision checked (and overall eye health examined) to find out if there are any issues with the eyes and vision. On rare occasion, both hearing and vision can be affected simultaneously (as was the case for famed Helen Keller). This has a very big impact on management of childhood hearing loss: when hearing loss is significant, supplementing understanding with visual cues (gestures, written information, ASL) becomes very important. If vision is challenged as well, it makes sense that listening and spoken language will be the communication modality, rather than ASL. Typically, a pediatric ophthalmologist (eye surgeon) is brought onto the team to give a full assessment of the health and function of the eyes. If there are visual acuity limitations, perhaps eyeglasses with corrective lenses are indicated to help the child see well. If the eyes check out normal, the ophthalmologist takes a back seat on the team, and remains available for ongoing checks, such as double-checking vision prior to the child starting kindergarten. When kids go to school, we need to make sure their vision hasn't changed and if so, help them to see well, to support learning to read and write.

The audiologist is tasked with the initial identification of the hearing loss, and ongoing testing to detail how much hearing the child has for the sake of fitting devices to help him or her hear better. The audiologist monitors hearing periodically, keeping an eye out for things like onset of ear infections, or a progression of sensorineural hearing loss. The audiologist communicates changes in hearing to the ENT physician (either due to ear health issues or a progression of the hearing loss) as this has medical implications for the ENT physician to address. In concert, progression/change in hearing has audiological implications for the audiologist to address. Adjustments to devices, addition of assistive technology (like FM systems, or visual alerts at home), and replacement of devices falls to the audiologist to manage with the family.

Perhaps the most obvious example of the team approach to family-centered management of childhood hearing loss is the CI team. Many of the major medical institutions that have a robust CI program have an established process for considering a child's candidacy for CI, considering the whole child. Often, it is the audiologist and/or ENT who identify if a child is a candidate for CI. If the child's hearing loss is severe enough to warrant consideration for CI, the ENT evaluates if the child is a candidate medically. Medical candidacy includes things like "is the child healthy enough to undergo an elective surgery?" and "is there a hearing nerve present?" (sometimes there isn't a nerve . . . that means CI isn't a viable approach, but there are other possible approaches, such as auditory brainstem implant). As part of the process for determining CI candidacy, the child should be evaluated by a developmental psychologist (sometimes referred to as a neuropsychologist). The purpose of seeing a neuropsychologist is to see where the child is in cognitive development, as well as language development, and if CI is developmentally appropriate. Part of the decision includes "What is the child's therapy plan after getting the implant?" Just getting the implant doesn't mean the child will learn what to do with it; hence, demonstrating there is access to intensive speech-language therapy and LSLS services is one way of satisfying the neuropsychology (and speech-language pathology) candidacy requirements for CI. Finally, on many CI teams, there is a Teacher of the Deaf/Hard-of-Hearing or Deaf advocate/ASL instructor. A holistic consideration of a child's CI candidacy includes the perspective of several professionals who have a stake in seeing the child be a successful communicator, and how the parents have come to the conclusion that spoken language, supported by CI, is their preferred method for teaching their child language.

THE ROLE OF BEHAVIORAL HEALTH CLINICIANS

An important note to raise, particular to the role of the developmental psychologist on the management team, is an acknowledgment of mental health care for the child with hearing loss. It is outrageously difficult to be a preteen and teenager. Many of us, as adults, think back to junior high and high school, and shudder. How much more difficult might it be to be different, use hearing aids or CIs, and perhaps have a speech pattern that is characteristic of a person with childhood hearing loss? Add to that, not only does hearing loss risk delays in speech-language development, but also social-emotional development. Navigating relationships with peers prior to and during puberty is hard enough . . . what about a child who continues to struggle with the isolation created by having hearing loss, and having difficulty with easy communication? Teenagers are at risk for mental health challenges. Period. I would urge parents to maintain an open dialogue with their preteen and teenage children about their relationships with peers and emotional struggles. Normalize those feelings of isolation and rejection by peers; meaning, be specific about rejection happening to you when you were growing up. Think about an adult relative or adult family friend your teenager admires, and relate a story where that admired adult struggled with peer relationships in high school. This kind of attention to emotional well-being can be uncomfortable for parents, but it's one of the most important roles a parent can play. And, seek the assistance of any member of your child's management team, but in particular, the psychologist. He or she has the education, training, and skills necessary to identify depression and anxiety, as well as other mental health conditions, and advise treatment. Depression and anxiety are extremely common in all teenagers, and teens with hearing loss are no exception.

THE PARENT-IN-CHIEF

It bears explicitly stating that the parents and child are the most integral members of the management team. The team surrounding the child with hearing loss are advisors, not the leaders. One analogy that is sometimes used to describe the role of clinicians is that parents are the president, and the team of clinicians is the president's cabinet. Running with this analogy: there is a secretary of state, secretary of defense, secretary of the treasury, and so on. These members of the cabinet advise the president, but it is the president's decision. Sometimes, the president follows the guidance of the cabinet member(s), and sometimes the president makes a decision contrary to the guidance of his or her advisors. The parent is not her child's otolaryngologist, audiologist, neuropsychologist, speech-language pathologist, or Teacher of the Deaf/Hard-of-Hearing (even if the parent happens to be one of these, we're parents first, and let a colleague be the professional). The parent is not supposed to be the expert in these technical areas: the parent is an expert in raising her child. As the child grows and matures, it's both terrifying and exhilarating to see the child start to take an active role in making decisions regarding the management of his hearing loss. If the child is able to take leadership of his hearing-loss management during teenage years, this is just a further expression of the child appropriately becoming independent of parents. The child becomes responsible for checking his hearing aid batteries, and making sure his earmolds are clean. The child becomes an advocate for himself in the classroom, asking the teacher to turn on the FM system microphone if the teacher forgets. The child seeks out friends who value him as an individual, and sees him not for his hearing loss, but as someone who is interesting and unique. The challenge for parents, of course, is to let the child take on leadership responsibility for his own hearing-loss management team. This isn't so different from a parent allowing any child to decide when to get an after-school job, buy a car, and start paying for her car insurance. Getting from newborn with newly diagnosed hearing loss to independent, balanced, emotionally stable young adult is a testament to human resilience. My children are still too young for me to have experienced the pride of seeing them strike their own paths in life, but I'm looking forward to that day. How much sweeter would it be for the parents of a child with hearing loss?

8

EXPERIENCES AND PRACTICAL ADVICE

All the background information about diagnostic tests, assistive devices, and educational plans is important information. But what about the actual day-to-day of being a child with hearing loss, or being the parent of a child with hearing loss? This chapter can really only touch on a few aspects of the influence of hearing loss on a child's world. Every child and family is different, and the struggles and triumphs are unique to each person. So, this chapter tries to offer some basic perspectives on how living with hearing loss makes some aspects of plotting one's course in the world different, and sometimes harder. There are a couple themes that are used to make the point, and are included because of their sheer importance: parent-to-parent connections and bullying. Without a doubt, not every challenge can be anticipated, and it's okay when parents get caught off guard. Parents of children with normal hearing and no other developmental issues are caught off guard routinely by life's challenges, so why should it be any different for parents of children with hearing loss? Thankfully, children are highly resilient, and as long as the bare minimum needs are met (including unconditional love), kids manage and succeed. To that end, the behavioral health (mental well-being) is given attention here as well: the behavioral health of the child, you the parent, and other siblings. This chapter wraps up with examples of what parents have done to help themselves and their families make their way through a world that includes childhood hearing loss.

It's tough being a young child. With every stage, there are challenges that are confusing. When the child is an infant, there's awesome snuggles and warmth and new and interesting things that happen constantly, but also these pains in the tummy that happen every couple hours that are only relieved when the child is fed. Why don't my parents know this is going to happen and stop it!? Sometimes, there are other pains in the belly that only subside when I burp (and spit up all over the place) or when I fart. It's exhausting being an infant. It doesn't get any easier as a toddler, either. All these big people around me move faster than I can, they can reach those shiny things I want and aren't giving me, they control the food, and turn off that screen that shows me my cartoons and say "that's enough screen time." At least I can get them to read the same book, over and over, until I decide that's enough and I'm bored. Preschoolers are pretty mobile, and very curious: there's a bunch of cool things under the sink in the kitchen (cleaning supplies) and in the toolbox in the basement (e.g., the utility knife). People also keep asking me to keep my voice down when my little sister is napping, which is really frustrating, because how am I supposed to remember every time she's asleep? And there's this new thing called "time out" that I do *not* like very much at all. Eventually, though, a child is able to start putting some complex thoughts together, and telling parents all about what's important to them. Being heard feels really good (although sometimes there's not enough hours in the day to hear everything the child wants to say). The child going into kindergarten, and over the next couple years, really starts to understand things like "cause and effect." If I tell a lie and get caught, I'm going to lose a privilege (or worse, no dessert). If I say "please" and "thank you" I get praise, so I'm going to keep doing that. This more sophisticated, cause-effect navigation of the world sets the stage for formal education to begin. Language is based on the rules of cause and effect, and is the most effective way for the brain to start putting together really complex thoughts. One of the earliest and most focused efforts at the start of elementary school is based on children developing mastery of language: this comes from establishing preliteracy and early literacy skills (reading and writing). Literacy sets the stage for all education that progresses from elementary school, forward.

Supporting the child with hearing loss from infancy through early elementary-school age requires love, patience, and language. Love is something that is programmed into our DNA, so that's a given. Patience: well, parents have more or less of that, and children teach us the limits of our patience. Language, on the other hand, is not a given. Most often, in children with normal hearing, language comes along at a reasonable pace. Sometimes children with no hearing loss or other developmental challenges need help learning language (I've seen estimates that 10 percent of the time, toddlers are speech delayed), and those who don't get help sometimes have language challenges that extend through childhood. Since language isn't guaranteed to come in on time without help anyway, consider the hit-or-miss access to language that happens when hearing isn't something easy to do. CIs really make words come front and center for a child who otherwise has essentially no hearing, but when there's some distance between the child with CIs and the person that child is supposed to listen to, the words don't always come through clearly. When there's background noise, the same happens: words drop out and it's hard to piece together the meaning. The same can be assumed when a child uses hearing aids. Consistent quiet, structured time, with activities geared toward language development, might help to make up for the missed opportunities to overhear language during the rest of the day. If this "quiet language-activity time" happens often enough for years, the child with hearing loss might build a large enough vocabulary, supporting a well-developed sense of "self" and ability to navigate the complex world of friends and family. Being able to navigate one's world without immediately resorting to protection from a parent means the child has attained a level of independence, which breeds confidence. These are vital qualities in a child who has his work cut out for him as he makes his way from elementary school to adulthood.

PARENT-TO-PARENT CONNECTIONS

A constant theme throughout this book is "How do we combat the isolation caused by childhood hearing loss?" The statistics indicate that childhood hearing loss is the most common permanent health condition that is present at birth. It affects roughly one in every 250 children (in developed countries; it's even more common in the developing world). And yet, most parents do not know any other children with hearing loss, or adults who had hearing loss from a young age. The diagnosis of hearing loss in a young child seems like a threat to the child's well-being, a threat the parent guards against like a mother bear over her cubs. Who could possibly understand the emotions a parent feels when having to face this threat to his or her child? Certainly not the audiologist. Certainly not the ENT. But another parent who has a child with hearing loss would.

No two kids are alike, and no two parents' experiences with their children are alike. But there is a common bond shared by all parents of children with hearing loss. Conveyed to me by one father: "Everyone who is part of the Hard-of-Hearing community has full privilege to talk with anyone else with a CI or has hearing aids." Parents have described being on vacation and running into another family who has a child with hearing aids or CIs. They immediately hit it off, end up sharing the rest of vacation together, children between the families quickly become playmates, and viola: there's a lifelong friendship between complete strangers. What two families would otherwise immediately become so friendly? In New England, where I live, unfamiliar people just don't talk with one another besides the very occasional, and very reserved, "Hello." But these open invitations to conversation are commonplace between families who have kids with hearing loss. In this, it seems hearing loss is anti-isolating: it opens the door to a vibrant community of people who share a common bond.

One of the first, and most important, connections to make when a child is diagnosed with hearing loss is with another parent who has had these similar experiences. It is commonplace in a facility with a large audiology staff for an email to go out to the team: "Anyone have on their caseload a child with moderately severe hearing loss and dad is a first responder?" Someone knows someone who has a family that fits the bill. Parent-to-parent connections are more important than the advice from a team of highly educated clinicians who have never "been there" in person. This is a special club, and only the cool kids are invited.

Parent support groups exist online and in person. Social media (like blogs, discussion groups, and Facebook) is amazing at bringing people together with similar interests and experiences from anywhere in the world. The Internet can be a scary place, filled with misinformation and online bullies, but it can also be comforting as well. I'll spend a little time on social media later in this chapter, but let's start with face-to-face connections. This may seem old fashioned in the age of constant digital connection, but it's hard to get a hug from someone through the computer.

A staple of family-centered intervention for children with hearing loss is connecting parents with a "Parent-Infant Group" in their community. Participation in these groups sometimes is geared toward developmental stimulation for the child with hearing loss, but there is the added benefit of parents getting to know one another. Setting the stage for parent-to-parent interaction is not an accident! Often, these are playgroups for children with hearing loss and are associated with schools for the deaf and hard-of-hearing, university programs, and even audiology and ENT practices. One amazing example of a community support program geared toward parents is Hear My Dreams (http://www.hearmydreams.com).[1] This parent-to-parent support group meets every other month, as well as once a year for a summer picnic. Hear My Dreams was founded by and is facilitated by audiologist Megan Ford, AuD, and is affiliated with her private audiology practice in Littleton, Massachusetts. I had the pleasure of meeting with parents who participate in Hear My Dreams as I gathered information for this book. Even though I don't qualify to be a member (I am not the parent of a child with hearing loss), I enjoyed it thoroughly and hope to be invited to join again sometime! It is very affirming to hear others who have struggled with something that you, yourself, have struggled with. Being able to share your own personal struggles, and be heard, was described by one parent as one of the most uplifting experiences of her life.

During a support-group meeting, parents describe both the joys of raising a child with hearing loss, as well as the pain of what is different. This is an opportunity to unload some powerful emotions in a safe environment, where everyone follows the same ground rules! Everything from a debrief of an emotionally painful experience with parents who "get it," to practical advice from other parents about the quirks of raising a child with hearing loss. Appointments with the ENT, audiologist, or speech-language pathologist might be cathartic for parents on occasion, when some big emotions are unpacked during the visit, but that's not the most common place where parents really open up. And that's understandable, since "doctors' offices" aren't always the most relaxing places. Healthcare providers are honored to be able to be emotionally present with families when we are needed that way, but it's not an expectation that parents feel this comfortable with us. If you are lucky enough to have more than one support group in your area, check them all out: maybe one is more convenient for you, but the other offers different and helpful contacts. Join if you can, but know there is no obligation (you have enough on your plate). This is part of taking-care-of-you.

Whether the support group is a developmental playgroup for the children, and parents connect informally, or the group is specifically geared to be parent-to-parent, there are a few important characteristics of an effective support group. There need to be "ground rules" that are understood and followed by all. These rules relate to confidentiality, respect for differing opinions, and being present in the moment (i.e., not checking emails and texts while someone is opening up). It is optimal when the group is facilitated by someone knowledgeable about hearing loss and children: this could be a parent who has an older child with hearing loss and this parent-facilitator has "been there, done that" and can be a role model for other parents; this could be an audiologist, psychologist, or speech-language pathologist; this could be a social worker or ENT physician, or perhaps a deaf adult, or a hearing adult whose parents are deaf. The facilitator is helpful then both as a moderator and as a resource to answer those questions that are of general interest to the group, and not a healthcare-related question specific to a particular child.

SUPPORTING YOURSELF AND CHILD THROUGH LIFE'S CHALLENGES

Supporting your child (and yourself and the rest of the family) through life's changing landscape is impressively difficult, and challenges posed by hearing loss often amplify the difficulties. The mantra throughout this book has been about helping to support language development, because lagging language development complicates so many of life's hurdles, from the trivial to the monumental. Here's a few examples to illustrate experiences that can be complicated by communication barriers.

Imagine having a two-and-a-half-year-old who has hearing loss and got CIs when he was just over one year old. He is making good strides in language development but still has a way to go for his language to be on par with other kids his age. His audiologist and speech language pathologist judge that by his current progress, he will catch up to his peers when he hits kindergarten, so he is on track to go to the local (mainstream) public school. He uses a few baby signs to facilitate wants and needs (used most often when he is too upset to use words). And his mother is pregnant and is due soon. How do you communicate something so complex and life-changing with the two-and-a-half-year-old with hearing loss and language delays? How do you prepare your toddler for the arrival of a new baby? Guaranteed, there are parents in support groups who have been in those shoes and can help navigate that one.

Here's another example that was relayed to me by a parent: the mother of a preschool-aged girl with hearing loss is stay-at-home, until her husband is laid off from his job, and she has to go back to work while he finds another job. In the meantime, though, the father will be taking care of his daughter, taking her to gymnastics, playgroups, and speech-language therapy sessions. His daughter communicates using both ASL and spoken language, although her speech is tough to understand unless you are very familiar with her. When she gets frustrated and can't get her point across, she tantrums, big time. Dad picked up some ASL, although not nearly as much as Mom, since he was working outside the home and she was home with their daughter. Mom also understands their daughter's speech pretty well, but Dad has a tough time. How do these parents cope with the stress of the potential financial and personal upheaval, while managing a potentially profound communication barrier between Dad and his daughter, now that the two of them are going to have to figure each other out?

Here's an all-too-common crisis that most parents can relate to: a parent has a couple young children, and they go into a department store, and one of the kids wanders off and the parent is freaked out trying to find them, terrified their child has been kidnapped. In this particular event (shared with me by one father) the older child (age four years) is a boy with hearing loss who has a CI in one ear, hearing aid in the other, and the younger sibling is his two-year-old sister with normal hearing. The two-year-old sister is in and out of the child seat in the shopping cart, and the four-year-old boy is walking beside them. At some point, the little girl demands to hold onto something she shouldn't have and Dad has to negotiate it away from her and deal with her losing her temper. While this is happening, the little boy wanders off to look at something in another aisle. Dad finally scoops up his wailing daughter, sticks her in the cart and they push forward. Dad goes only about ten feet and looks to see where his son is. And doesn't see him. And calls for him. And there's no answer. And then looks down the nearest couple aisles, and doesn't see him. His daughter is still whining about not getting to keep the thing Dad took away from her. Fast-forward: with no luck finding his son quickly, Dad sprinted to the front of the store and found a manager who locked the store down and all employees swept the store looking for the boy. The little boy was found within a few minutes, wandering around looking for his dad and little sister, in no distress, just trying to figure out how he would find them. With the usual department store noise of other carts, music played over the store's speakers, and parents and noisy children, the little boy couldn't hear his father (even though he was probably pretty close by when his dad first called for him), and both Dad and son happened to walk away from, rather than toward, each other when Dad started looking for him. And with the racks of clothes, shelves, and so on, they couldn't see each other. Of course, this can happen with any parent, but his son's hearing loss and inherent difficulty hearing and localizing his dad's voice from any distance at all made it easier for it to happen in the first place, and harder to resolve.

Those are just three real examples that give some idea what is meant by "life's challenges," and I'm sure you can come up with a number of others: such as the family relocating; the death of a grandparent; a health crisis in the family; divorce. These circumstances are challenging for all families, and when we are faced with them, open and clear communication helps to manage the circumstances. So, if there is a communication barrier between the child and parents, how much more difficult is it to prepare the child for life's changes, and help the child cope and adjust?

SUPPORTING YOUR CHILD'S SOCIAL-EMOTIONAL DEVELOPMENT AND NEGOTIATING PEER RELATIONSHIPS IN SCHOOL

Several times throughout this book, and in this chapter, I've touched on social-emotional development being at risk when a child has hearing loss. Put very simply, is this child happy? Does he make friends with children his age, and does he become familiar with adults and then interact with them? Does he exhibit confidence? Or does he seem unhappy? Is he socially isolated, finding it challenging and too scary to try to make friends? Does he cling to a single caregiver, and show more than the usual stranger anxiety? In truth, many children who are typically developing "come out of their shell" at different times. Some children are just shy by nature. Lagging in social-emotional development due to hearing loss is more than just being shy. Children learn, with experience, to self-soothe. This self-soothing is something infants do: sometimes with a pacifier, sometimes with a fist, and sometimes they just decide they've cried enough and choose to stop now. As we get older, we might talk about "centering" ourselves or "getting ourselves in the right frame of mind." Simply put, it's de-stressing by choice. Being able to self-soothe is a very important social-emotional skill, as it helps the child to become a team with her parent in raising her. Being a parent is exhausting, and that exhaustion is beyond description when you have a baby who is colicky (which is the epitome of not being able to self-soothe).

Children who are making good strides cognitively, who are curious and whose brains are eager to learn new things but who are lagging in language can easily become frustrated by their lack of ability to express themselves and advocate for themselves with caregivers. When communication is routinely unsuccessful, this creates a pattern of stress in the child. He might come to expect conflict with a caregiver who is at her wits end trying to figure out what her child wants. The expectation of conflict turns into full-blown behavioral challenges, like tantrums and aggressive behavior (toward himself in self-injurious behaviors, or aggression toward others). I recall a patient of mine who was adopted from another country at age two years, and was found to have significant hearing loss. International adoptees are sometimes developmentally delayed, and this is not surprising, given there is often a lack of developmental stimulation in their environment, such as in an orphanage. It is typical in the Boston area for international adoptees to go through a battery of developmental assessments in the months after they come home with their new parents, and hearing evaluation is part of that battery. This particular child was found to have moderately severe hearing loss in both ears. His behavior was extremely challenging, to the point his parents were constantly on guard, as he could easily injure himself. Over time, he did develop language, and with increasingly sophisticated language his behavior became more manageable.

But along that path to manageable behavior, this child was diagnosed with Oppositional Defiant Disorder and his management included psychotherapy and family therapy, in addition to ASL instruction and intensive speech-language therapy. Of course, this extreme case is used for illustration. There were biological and environmental factors at play with this child, and despite such significant early challenges, the family found their stride, and their child was in a mainstream public school program last I worked with them. The point to this story is to make use of the resources available to your child, and attend to behavioral health/ mental health challenges with the same priority as early speech-language evaluation and therapy.

Children diagnosed with hearing loss in the first few months of life typically develop very close ties with family, since members of the family are known before any lack of language makes a family member a "stranger." Newborns get to know their family through touch and smell; babies don't even see three feet in front of them clearly until they are about three to four months old. All the closeness and skin-to-skin contact is extremely effective nonverbal communication with a young infant. That closeness continues well into childhood. Of course, the toddler years are challenging for nearly every child, as they have fits and spurts of needing to express themselves better than their language skills allow. If a child with hearing loss has a need to express himself that is far beyond his language abilities, this mismatch between need and ability breeds lots of frustration. As a child's expressive language abilities advance, the frustration lessens. Getting through those toddler years is like running a gauntlet: sometimes families make it through unscathed. But it's a tough path. So what happens when a child hits preschool and finds it really difficult to communicate with normal-hearing peers? What if his speech patterns have distortions that make it hard for people unfamiliar with him to understand what he's saying? What if a new playmate wants him to do something, but he isn't able to follow (due to limited language, or not yet benefiting to his full potential with hearing aids or CIs)? That playmate might move along with other activities and play with other children rather than continue trying to engage with the child with hearing loss. All things being equal, children with hearing loss do very well with children with normal hearing, where the child with normal hearing can act as a language mentor. But it's also very good for a child with hearing loss to meet other children with hearing loss. Some of the best playgroups are ones that have a mix of children with hearing loss and children with normal hearing, with those children with more advanced language serving as peer role models.

Parents have described their own anxieties that pertain to their child's social-emotional development, and strategies they've used that have worked so far. One mother described a real challenge helping her infant learn to self-soothe. Noah has severe-to-profound hearing loss and he was seven months old when I met him and his parents. Self-soothing was a problem at bedtime, since the usual soft soothing voice to calm a baby, or white noise machine, weren't something that Noah could hear. When the lights were turned off, he was really cut off from the parent putting him to bed. Some recommendations: follow the same bedtime routines as you would for any child (still sing songs, for instance, but hold the baby against you while singing so they are soothed by your vibrations), but never have the room completely dark. A good nightlight is a must (one that isn't too bright, but certainly not too weak). Some children sleep best with blackout shades; in fact, a child sleep therapist I know is a very strong proponent to help children get adequate sleep, especially during summer months when there are actually too many hours of daylight. But for children with hearing loss, think twice about blackout shades, since these children rely more heavily on light to have a sense of their environment. A benefit of having a baby with hearing loss? It's not so imperative to have everyone in the house tiptoe around after the baby goes down for a nap or is put to bed for the night. Short of stampeding children causing enough floor vibration to shake the child's bed, older siblings can just play without fear of waking their little brother.

When a child with hearing loss who uses hearing aids or CIs is in a mainstream school setting, she is usually the only child in her class who uses devices to hear better. In early elementary-school years, peers are often very curious, and in fact have a positive attitude toward their classmate with the neat devices. Their honest, unfiltered questions about the devices and what makes their classmate different is refreshing. It's pretty easy to "normalize" the hearing loss and devices to children this age: in general, younger elementary-school-aged children readily accept peers with different abilities as part of the normal way of things. These differences do become much more challenging, though, as children grow older and the social pecking order is getting established, and individuals feel the competition to rank as high as possible. Differences can easily be exploited to devalue the person with a physical challenge so that another can rise up in the ranks of popularity. It's cruel, but it seems to be programmed into our DNA; check out the literature on theories of social organization, and you'll see that nearly every social mammal (including humans) arranges their peer groups according to a pecking order.

While it's easy to normalize differences to the whole class, it can be challenging for a child with hearing loss to easily make new friends with classmates. First of all, it can be difficult for a person with hearing loss to hear and understand new people (such as the child meeting his or her classmates for the first time). When children get involved in a group activity or group play, they typically have rapid verbal exchange, and talk over one another. For the child with hearing loss, being able to keep up with who is talking, and what was said, can be pretty overwhelming. Not keeping up with who said what means he can't be as engaged. This risks the child being able to make friends with his playmates. One way to help facilitate a child with hearing loss making friends: parents arranging one-on-one playdates early in the school year, with a few of their child's different classmates. See which classmates hit it off with their child, let a friendship develop organically, and then build the number of children joining for playdates. And, of course, make playdates with other children with hearing loss (hopefully, families who met at Parent-Infant group are able to stay in touch, even as the children get older).

Work with the teacher and special-education personnel (Teacher of the Deaf and Hard-of-Hearing, speech-language pathologist) to create opportunities for children to work on projects one on one, rather than always in bigger groups where it can be easy for the child with hearing loss to get lost. The child with hearing loss should be encouraged to be vocal about his or her needs, such as asking only one person talk at a time, and that it's okay to ask people to repeat themselves. Friendly assertiveness is an excellent trait to develop for someone who will need to advocate for himself/herself socially, educationally, and occupationally. If the child with hearing loss is agreeable to the idea, work with teachers to bring the topic of hearing loss into the classroom curriculum, such as during health or science education, or even social studies and history. There is a very rich history of Deaf culture in the United States, such as the fact that so many people who lived on Martha's Vineyard (an island off the coast of Massachusetts) in the 1800s were deaf, that in the island town of Chilmark, people were required to know sign language in order to settle there.[2] Another opportunity to build hearing-loss topics into the curriculum: Alexander Graham Bell actually considered himself a teacher of the deaf, more than an inventor and scientist, and his wife was born with hearing loss. Bell invented the telephone in an effort to help people with hearing loss communicate with the wider hearing world. The "decibel" is named in honor of A. G. Bell, and (as we know) is abbreviated "dB," or one-tenth of a Bel (a unit of sound intensity).[3]

Of the children I have managed audiologically in my fifteen years as an audiologist, I would estimate that 50 percent of those aged nine to eighteen years were picked on at least once for having hearing loss and using hearing aids or CIs. It is so common that I would bring it up with parents when their child was in kindergarten to first grade to alert them to be on the lookout. From an audiologist's perspective, not only do I want my patients to be happy, healthy, well-adjusted people, but I want them to use their hearing aids! When a child with hearing loss is picked on for using his hearing aids, he might start refusing to put hearing aids on in the morning. Maybe he will put them on, but take them off once he gets on the bus, or get to school and is out of parents' line of sight. Kids can be creative and sneaky, but eventually, teachers will ask parents, "What's wrong with Jack's hearing aids? He told me they are broken," while coming home with hearing aids in (after being out of sight of the classmate who made him feel self-conscious for using hearing aids). When this behavior is detected, one of the most important things for a parent to do is to normalize the child's behavior, and do *not* punish him for not using hearing aids and lying about it. To do so would victimize him again, and threaten the safety he feels toward his parents. It is reasonable for a child to respond to social pressure by removing his or her hearing aids. It's the quickest and easiest way to remove the source of ridicule (well, not really, but this is the logic of the child). Rather than express anger, unhappiness, or even mother-bear protectiveness, ask, "Well, honey, hearing aids are how you hear your friends and teachers, so it's important you use them. How do we solve this problem with [offending classmate] being so mean and ignorant?" Be prepared for a silent shoulder shrug. And even though you, the parent, are most certainly going to take charge in this and discuss resolution with the school (reach out to the teacher and special-education director as a first step), approaching your child in a manner that welcomes his participation in the resolution shows that you respect him while showing it is necessary to "step up" and meet these conflicts head-on. And even though you will be taking charge, support your child in assisting with the conflict resolution. A parent's immediate reaction to their child being bullied is to "go medieval" on whoever was the perpetrator or was complicit. But being bullied is in large part about losing control. When a parent takes away what little control there was from the child being bullied, to the child, it feels like she is being victimized again.

Children and teenagers with hearing loss are at much higher risk for being bullied in school and online than their normal hearing peers. And their communication barrier can interfere with them getting help, which exacerbates the problem. Bullying is an unfortunately common occurrence in school-aged kids, and it starts at younger ages than one might expect.[4] According to www.stopbullying.gov, children as young as preschool report bullying with some regularity. While a preschooler's interpretation of "bullying" might be a very simplified one (for instance, a "bully" might be anyone he or she thinks is "not nice"), there is a common definition for true bullying. According to stopbullying.gov, bullying is "unwanted, aggressive behavior among school aged children that involves a real or perceived power imbalance. The behavior is repeated, or has the potential to be repeated, over time. Bullying includes actions such as making threats, spreading rumors, attacking someone physically or verbally, and excluding someone from a group on purpose" (quotation from http://www.stopbullying.gov/what-is-bullying/index.html).[5]

Junior high school is just awkward for everyone, and it's not surprising that bullying is most common in these grades. Children this age are going through a very typical process of finding their identity outside the family unit, which requires them to navigate relationships with peers that have all of a sudden become much more complex. It's much easier to navigate these troubled waters if you have a fantastic vocabulary and are very agile using it! Meaning, if one boy verbally teases another boy, the one being teased has a great chance at limiting future teasing if he is able to give a clever response. This kind of verbal sparring is normal adolescent/preadolescent behavior, and is part of kids establishing their social order. Put simply, kids can be mean. It is how they figure out who is "king of the hill" and who the popular kids are. What if the verbal sparring turns destructive? What if one student is singled out as the target of ridicule by another for the purpose of intimidation? This is bullying.

Is it necessary to be popular in school? It helps. Children with good relationships with peers experience less stress, show better attention to schoolwork, have better school attendance, and have less anxiety and depression. Children who are socially isolated are at higher risk for being bullied. Thankfully, school personnel have elevated their attention to building positive relationships among students; educators know that it's hard to live up to your academic potential if you're constantly worried about being picked on by classmates. And we're not just talking about innocent, good-natured "ribbing." Bullying is dangerous. Bullying escalates to physical violence regularly, and even if it doesn't, the emotional toll on the target of the aggression can be devastating. Tragically, there are occasional news reports of teenagers committing suicide as a result of bullying. If bullying is so common for all children, how much more likely is it for a child with hearing loss, whose social-emotional development is at risk? One of the best articles I've read on the topic of bullying of children with hearing loss was written by some brilliant pediatric audiologists, and can be found at http:// www.howsyourhearing.org/documents/bullying.pdf.[6] While this article was written for audiologists, it is an easy read and I encourage all parents of school-aged children with hearing loss to read it. Given the high likelihood of, at least, getting picked on and potentially things escalating to bullying, it makes sense to talk about this with your child in advance, and create a plan. Many schools have a formal bullying-response plan, thanks in part to a 2011 White House summit that identified bullying as more than a harmless "rite of passage." It would make sense to include in your child's IEP a plan to monitor for and respond to bullying, such as activating the school's established bullying-response plan. While schools bear responsibility for ensuring a safe environment, including this language specifically in the child's IEP elevates the school's vigilance.

There are excellent resources for parents to learn about bullying risk, prevention, and resolution: start with www.stopbullying.gov. School personnel have training in bullying prevention and management, and they often have materials they can share. Pediatricians and family-medicine physicians have deep understanding of bullying and can serve as an advocate for you and your child. Speech-language pathologists and social workers can be excellent resources for families, and often are identified as "safe adults" if they have been part of your child's IEP team. There are even specialized clinics to assist in bullying resolution, particularly in children with special needs. One such example is the Bullying and Cyberbullying Prevention and Advocacy Collaborative (BACPAC) at Boston Children's Hospital.[7] I've had a couple patients see the BACPAC clinical team, and am grateful they were able to assist with some tough situations. For more information about this program, see http://www.childrenshospital.org/centers-and-services/bullying-and-cyberbullying-prevention-and-advocacy-collaborative-bacpac-program.

SUPPORTING YOUR RELATIONSHIPS WITH YOUR CHILD BUT ALSO WITH FAMILY AND FRIENDS

Parents described the anxieties they felt in the months after their child was diagnosed with hearing loss, and these focused on anxiety about their child's future relationships. They didn't raise anxiety about grades, or jobs; the fears they expressed were about whether or not they would be able to get to know their child, and whether or not their child would face social isolation because of being different. One mother related, "Can I get to know her? I didn't love her any less, but I wondered 'who is going to communicate with her?' Now she's super gregarious." Another mother described an early anxiety for her child: "He's going to be so different from every other kid in the family." This family had lots of aunts, uncles, and cousins on both mom's and dad's side of the family, and family get-togethers are epic. One of the most profound and touching questions I've ever had a parent ask me came from a mother when I diagnosed her daughter with severe-to-profound hearing loss at age two years: "Does this mean she won't ever get married?!" I use this touching example of a mother's fear for her daughter's future with audiology students to help them understand the difference between a question seeking an academic answer (a "content" question) versus a question that is actually communicating profound emotions related to the parent's grief. Universally, parents described the best way to manage these feelings of anxiety is to get to know other families who have children with hearing loss. One father said, of his first experience joining a Parent-Infant playgroup, "They weren't deaf kids. They weren't hard-of-hearing kids. They were happy kids! They were rowdy kids!" In the playgroups, it's beneficial for there to be some older kids who are making great strides: parents of younger children are able to see tangible possibilities of what their child might be able to do. This breeds confidence. As a parent of one of those older kid with hearing loss said, "She's doing well. But she's doing well differently." Another parent strongly recommended finding a deaf babysitter. I have to admit, this isn't something I had ever thought of, but it makes great sense! The child sees his or her parents entrust his or her care to a responsible adult with hearing loss: this deaf adult is in a position of authority, and is a person to be trusted.

An elementary-school teacher with progressive hearing loss bravely shared some perspectives that fit right along with those of parents of young children. This teacher is very well respected in the community, and has adult children of her own. She has family members with hearing loss, so there is almost certainly a hereditary component to the hearing loss, and likely she was born with some degree of hearing loss. Despite there being a family history of childhood hearing loss, hers was only identified when she was seven or eight years old when her hearing was first screened in school. Her hearing loss was not discussed within her family, and her own feelings toward it were shaped by her experiences of what she could and couldn't do. She managed through school without using hearing aids or other assistive devices, but did find hearing challenging by the time she went to college. Now, her hearing loss is in the moderate range, and her relationship with her hearing loss has changed over the years. She has struggled to find a level of acceptance with the hearing loss, and described the challenges of being able to socialize with friends any time there is background noise (such as at a restaurant). She described feeling "outside" in these group settings, and "not really included" simply because she cannot effectively participate in spontaneous conversation in those noisier social settings. A few things this teacher said resonated deeply, based on her description of her successes but also her frustrations and difficulties with her relationship with her hearing loss: "Always treat your child as normal. They will be fine, just support them in their dreams, and use every possible tool to help them. Talk openly within the family, so they know this is never something to hide or be ashamed of. It's not who they are, it's what they have." The best way we can teach our children to love themselves, including *all* the things that make them who they are, is to openly and honestly acknowledge them, with their perfections and imperfections. Doing this helps them see themselves through your loving eyes, and teaches them they are "good enough" and worthy of love and respect exactly as they are.

Normal-hearing siblings of children with hearing loss are, of course, just as deserving of their parent's attention. And that can be a recipe for enormous guilt to pile onto the parents who are doing their best to just meet the needs of the child with hearing loss. There is real potential for resentment, which can be expressed as acting out and other challenging behaviors. If the sibling resents all the attention being given to her brother or sister with hearing loss this can disrupt the relationships in the family. It is quite common for an older sibling to either "fake" having a hearing loss, or just outright ask if she can get hearing aids too! This behavior is a good sign that the sibling is asking for some attention. This call for attention isn't a good thing or a bad thing, but it should be heard. But what are parents to do if they feel they are at their limit and can't be everything their children need from them at all times?! Recall it's not necessary to be supermom or superdad: it's not realistic and kids certainly don't need perfect parents.

A clinical social worker described to me some ways that parents build relationships with their kids, even when those parents don't have daily contact, such as parents who are divorced, deployed in the military, or travel for work.[8] It's about establishing routines of contact and special time. There can be periods of time when a child sees his parent only once every couple weeks, but the relationship continues to flourish. Carving out protected time with a child, even if that happens only once every two weeks, can be very successful in supporting the relationship, so long as it's a solid routine. That special, protected time should be something both the parent and child thoroughly enjoy, such as going to the zoo or to a movie, or having a "camp out" in the family room with sleeping bags and flashlights. Marking the "special time" on a calendar that the child keeps or has access to helps her develop patience and trust. If every other Saturday afternoon she goes with one parent to see a movie, and she sees this on the calendar on the wall in her bedroom, she won't ask constantly, "When will we go to the movies again?" if you can say every time, "Go look on your calendar and you'll see the answer for yourself." For a sibling of a child with hearing loss, having this occasional, but routine, solo contact with a parent is one suggestion that might work for a family.

But it's not just about the parents' relationship with normal-hearing siblings, there is a need to support the normal-hearing siblings' relationship with their brother or sister with hearing loss. And this can be tricky, especially if the child with hearing loss and the sibling with normal hearing don't easily access each other's language. For instance, if a normal-hearing sibling is in elementary school, and his little brother with hearing loss receives speech-language therapy and ASL instruction with his mother during the day, then the normal-hearing sibling is reliant on parents to teach him ASL so he can more effectively communicate with his little brother. If the parents are trying to figure it all out themselves, they will have a tough time being an ASL language model. A suggestion given to me by a family was to enlist the sibling's help: if the older sibling is reading, have him read books to his sibling with hearing loss. In elementary school, kids are typically given reading tasks as homework, such as "Read aloud to a parent or family member for at least ten minutes every night." Why not kill two birds with one stone? The normal-hearing child in second grade can easily spend ten minutes reading two books to his little brother with CIs. Some children's books are geared toward enhancing ASL vocabulary, so the older sibling can learn the signs that go along with each page of the book while reading the accompanying words out loud. Regardless of the approach to integrating siblings' experiences together, keeping communication open between members of the family is crucial. Children do best when they feel their emotions are respected, selfish as those may be sometimes. It's better for a child to verbalize feelings of anger and jealousy toward a sibling with special developmental needs than for those emotions to be kept bottled inside, festering. Appealing to the sibling's willingness to help, or be protective at school of their brother or sister with hearing loss gives the sibling a sense of purpose and responsibility. Keep the sibling informed of what's happening with their brother or sister with hearing loss (for instance, plans to proceed with CI surgery) using language that is appropriate for the sibling's age and ability to understand. And parents are encouraged to look to behavioral health specialists (mental health counselors) sooner than later, if there is a disruption in the family's relationships.

STRIKING A BALANCE AND SUPPORTING YOURSELF AND YOUR RELATIONSHIPS

Parents of children with hearing loss have expressed a heightened sense of protectiveness of their child. Despite the fact that early identification and intervention for hearing loss brings about so much good, the experience of diagnosis, including the myriad medical tests and upheaval in life, and all that goes into effective intervention can be downright traumatic for parents. This stays with a parent forever. Most parents can recall specific details about the day their child was diagnosed with hearing loss. Things like the weather on that day, the color of the walls in the exam room, and where they parked their car when they went to the appointment. When powerful emotions accompany an event, our brains hang onto strange details, as though these random details might prove important and the brain wants to take note of them, just in case. Because we love our children so much, hearing something is "wrong" is a threat to our core being. So we go into protection mode. Would parents be so protective if the child didn't have hearing loss, or other challenges? Is this lingering need to be protective influencing whether or not you let your child engage in normal risk-taking activities? Just like any child who is otherwise typically developing, the child with hearing loss is going to do some things that get him into trouble, result in a broken bone or stitches, or get his heart broken. Certainly, not all parents who have experienced a diagnosis of childhood hearing loss become "helicopter parents" but I expect it is a conscious decision these parents make. It certainly is understandable if they are, but it's more helpful to moderate the overprotectiveness. That father who shared with me the story of losing his son in the department store: how could he ever again bring himself back to a normal level of vigilance?

While parents are advocating for their child's needs, it is easy for them to pay no attention to their own needs. Being told your beautiful newborn has hearing loss is devastating for many parents, and a cascade of grief ensues. One mother described "always trying to be strong for my daughter" and not showing anger or sadness, until she realized she was suppressing these important and valid emotions. Stifling the emotional reactions to a painful situation doesn't do a parent any favors! And while the parent is experiencing these powerful emotions, there are often multiple medical appointments, which adds to the stress and taxes parents' reserves. Oh, and do this while the baby is waking up every two hours to feed and parents are sleep deprived. If this is a first child, parents are trying to figure out how to take care of this needy little thing, and may feel overwhelmed just being a new parent, much less a new parent of a child with hearing loss. To top all this off, the mother's hormones (which peaked during pregnancy) are now plummeting, and there is a strong probability she will experience some level of postpartum depression. The fact parents survive this phase is a testament to human resilience.

Mothers and fathers commonly react differently to the diagnosis of hearing loss. Perhaps this is because men are socialized to show their emotions less, or perhaps it's an innate gender difference. Often, dads go into "fix it" mode and push to have every test done immediately, hearing aids on and the child fast-tracked for CIs, and stay up all hours of the night researching hearing-loss treatments. Moms often reach out to their closest friends or relatives and have some really good cries. The differences in how parents deal with their feelings of grief can easily create conflict. The way one parent expresses his or her grief might make it appear he or she is not emotionally available to their partner. If parents don't feel like they are "on the same page" with each other, and explicitly make it a point to be emotionally accessible, each can feel isolated, like they are going through this ordeal alone. These kinds of life-altering experiences can test a marriage. It is commonly accepted that divorce rates are higher in families who have children with special needs compared to families who have typically developing children. Alternatively, this might create a stronger bond between parents than they would have otherwise known. Stresses like this can be polarizing events: either parents become tighter than they would have otherwise, or they split apart. While not all marriages should necessarily be kept going, all things being equal, parenting is easier when both parents are able to communicate effectively with each other and are active participants in meeting the child's needs. This is true whether parents are together in a relationship or not. But if the marriage dissolves, communication between parents about their child is often far more difficult. Parents often described having to put their marriage "on hold" while addressing the immediate needs following the hearing loss diagnosis. When parents have a good enough communication that they can say this outright to each other, there are a lot less hurt feelings than if the marriage being put on hold sneaks up on both parents. To be clear, I'm not suggesting a person's marriage needs to go on autopilot because of childhood hearing loss, but marriage is easier on some days, harder on others. If all attention truly needs to focus on the child, both parents being on the same page means they go forward as a team. Really good teams also allow one parent to grieve and cope differently. Sometimes that means one parent shoulders the responsibilities for a short time until the other can reengage. Often, one parent takes the lead role in managing the appointments and interventions. If this is what works for your family, come to that decision jointly (rather than it being a reality that sneaks up on you). Sometimes it's obvious who should "take point" but consider this can be a burden to the one who shoulders the responsibility. Regardless how parents cope, if the relationship becomes threatened, use the resources available to you (just as you would with your child): individual and/or couples counseling is encouraged, and should be sought very early if there is communication breakdown, rather than waiting to see if problems will "fix themselves."

What about extended family relationships, and those with friends? Parents interviewed in preparation of this book reported that after telling extended family and friends of their child's hearing loss, they said things like "everyone knew someone with hearing loss—it's like they were coming out of the woodwork." One parent described her dread going to a family reunion *the day after* her young infant was diagnosed with permanent hearing loss. How was she going to tell people? Would she tell anyone? How would she hold her emotions in check? Parents described to me that reactions from family and friends were generally very supportive, with some surprising jewels of strength that would come from unexpected acquaintances. And there were obvious challenges, such as the "helpful" mother-in-law who seems to have solutions to every problem, no matter how little she knows about it. Family dynamics are tricky. One mother of a little boy (seven months old at the time of writing) described the difficulties she was encountering with her extended family: her son has a moderate degree of hearing loss, with some better hearing in the low pitches. So, he hears his name and many environmental sounds, with and without his hearing aids. Extended family observe his reactions and have gone so far as to say "See, he doesn't *really* need those hearing aids, does he?" Consequently, these are the same family members who tried to talk this mom, who has done exclusive breastfeeding of her son, that she should supplement his feedings with formula. Opinions are like a certain orifice; everybody has one.

Many of us have an online community of family and friends and we keep track of each other's lives with posts and status updates. People who move across the country from where they grew up can keep tabs on high-school friends, and it's easier to reconnect when we meet up at high-school reunions. Very often, people use online media to alert their extended network of friends and family of big life changes: engagement, pregnancy, and the birth of a child are favorites. One family I spoke with used Facebook to notify their extended friends and family of their child's hearing-loss diagnosis. They made phone calls to immediate family and a few close friends, and then wrote a carefully worded post, so that the majority of people they knew would all hear the news at about the same time. Not every family chooses to notify their world this way. But it is one way, and it means most people with whom parents interact will find out the news, so that parents don't have to repeat their story over and over. But just as with family who are full of opinions, online posts sometimes invite comments that are unwelcome. I've seen some awful comments on YouTube and marvel at the audacity of some people to be antagonistic. But then, usually it's easy enough to realize whoever posts such awful things must be thoroughly unloved. Good thing that's not us, or our kids.

FINAL THOUGHTS

How does a parent help their child with hearing loss navigate the trials and tribulations of growing up without being too overprotective? Much the same as all parents: messily. You are going to screw up. Your child will, someday, say "I hate you!" But she won't mean it, and she might even apologize later when she gets her temper under control. Several parents have shared stories that in the heat of an argument, their children pulled out their hearing aids or CIs, so they could end the argument, on their terms! Those who use ASL shut their eyes and shout "I can't hear you!" Talk about cutting you off! It is never a requirement for parents to be "perfect" at raising their child. Perfection is a falsehood: there is no such thing. And it is not necessary to be any more adept at parenting when your child has hearing loss (that is, it's not necessary to be supermom or superdad). Many parents, early in the process of grieving the news their child has hearing loss, have described feeling overwhelmed and incapable of giving their child what he or she needs. "Inadequacy" was a very common theme describing the emotions parents feel when they are hit with all the literature that says things like "Children need to start intensive language therapy from age six months or else they'll never catch up!" (that's not actually what the literature says, but it's easy for a parent to interpret it that way). These feelings of inadequacy might be coming on the tail of feelings of guilt. One mother told me that right after her daughter's diagnosis, she tallied up the times when she forgot to take her prenatal vitamins, and recalled "I had a glass of wine once." These feelings of guilt and inadequacy are no surprise: of course a parent would feel these feelings! The fact that *so* many parents report the same emotions shows us that this is a normal reaction to an abnormal situation. Parents feel guilt and inadequacy despite being actually in no way responsible for their child's hearing loss and prove to be far above "adequate" in raising their child. Since these emotions (or whatever other emotions you feel) are normal, there is no need to "fix" them. They are uncomfortable. They oftentimes get in the way of enjoying some of the things about having a baby: their funny noises, their touch, their smell. But it's possible to respect these negative emotions, and allow them to exist in you, while at the same time be present and enjoy your baby's funny noises, and how your baby feels and smells when he or she falls asleep on you. Those negative emotions will run their course, and they don't deserve the focus of your attention to the exclusion of all there is to enjoy about your child. When in Holland, smell the tulips.

UNDERSTANDING CHILDHOOD HEARING LOSS

This list of resources is not intended to be exhaustive, but to offer a breadth of content as a starting point and to supplement information made available from local audiologists and state organizations.

Referrals to Professions

- A consumer website hosted by the American Academy of Audiology www.HowsYourHearing.org: consumer-oriented information about hearing and hearing loss in adults and children. Searchable database to find an audiologist near you.
- American Board of Audiology: find a board certified audiologist with a specialty in pediatric audiology http://www.boardofaudiology.org/pediatric-audiology-specialty-certification/ or a specialty in cochlear implants http://www.boardofaudiology.org/cochlear-implant-specialty-certification/.
- Early Hearing Detection and Intervention—Pediatric Audiology Links to Services www.ehdi-pals.org: Find audiology facilities, resources about hearing, early intervention, and other helpful websites.

Educational Audiology

- Compendium of information by pioneering educational audiologist Karen Anderson, PhD available at https://successforkidswithhearingloss.com/
- Including material for the SIFTER and scoring the SIFTER:
- https://successforkidswithhearingloss.com/uploads/SIFTER.pdf
- https://successforkidswithhearingloss.com/uploads/SIFTER_Manual.pdf

National Associations for People Who Are Deaf or Hard-of-Hearing

- Alexander Graham Bell Associationhttp://www.listeningandspokenlanguage.org/: an association focusing on listening and spoken language approach to management of childhood hearing loss, they offer advocacy, education, research, and financial aid.
- National Association for the Deafhttp://nad.org/: an association with broad advocacy goals for the inclusion of the deaf in society. The use of ASL is a core value for NAD.
- Hearing Loss Association of Americahttp://www.hearingloss.org/: an advocacy group that seeks to improve communication access for all people with hearing loss by influencing public policy, increasing public awareness, and impacting how services are delivered to people with hearing loss.

Bullying Resources

- www.stopbullying.gov
- http://www.howsyourhearing.org/documents/bullying.pdf
- http://www.childrenshospital.org/centers-and-services/bullying-and-cyberbullying-prevention-and-advocacy-collaborative-bacpac-program

Informational Resources

Departments of public health, universal newborn hearing-screening programs have resources:

- The Massachusetts program websitewww.mass.bog/dph/ newbornhearingscreening: helpful links, family stories, speech and language developmental milestones.
- Federation for Children with Special Needswww.fcsn.org: thorough resources about IDEA and advocating for a child with special needs.
- Individuals with Disabilities Education Act websitehttp://idea.ed. gov/: detailed information about Individuals with Disabilities Education Act, including early intervention (IFSP) and school-based services (IEP).
- State Commissions for the Deaf and Hard-of-Hearing. The example in Massachusetts is a highly organized, successful program. Their website has a remarkable amount of user-friendly information:http://www.mass.gov/eohhs/gov/departments/mcdhh/
- Signing Timeswww.signingtime.com: award-winning sign-language products, instructional DVDs and books, material geared toward different ages (included potty training, zero to three years, pre-K, etc.)
- Centers for Disease Control and Preventionhttp://www.cdc.gov/ ncbddd/hearingloss/documents/mild_uni_ref_list-updated_1-29-08.pdf: extensive list of references to scientific publications about mild and unilateral hearing loss.

Examples of a Local and National Parent Support Groups

- Hear My Dreamshttp://www.hearmydreams.com: facilitated and hosted in a private audiology practice.
- Hands and Voiceshttp://www.handsandvoices.org/: a nonprofit, parent-driven organization dedicated to supporting families of children who are deaf or hard of hearing. They are nonbiased about commu-

nication methodologies and believe that families can make the best choices for their child if they have access to good information and support.

- Parent to Parent USAwww.P2Pusa.org: emotional and informational support for families of children who have special needs. National Parent Connection (particularly for families who have a child with multiple disabilities).

NOTES

1. WELCOME TO HOLLAND . . . A CLINICIAN'S PERSPECTIVE

1. Emily Pearl Kingsley, "Welcome to Holland," *www.our-kids.org*, 1987, www.our-kids.org/Archives/Holland.html.

2. Fred H. Bess and Jack L. Paradise, "Universal Screening for Infant Hearing Impairment: Not Simple, Not Risk Free, Not Necessarily Beneficial, and Not Presently Justified," *Pediatrics* 93 (1994): 330–34.

3. Melody Harrison and Jackson Roush, "Age of Suspicion, Identification, and Intervention for Infants and Young Children with Hearing Loss: A National Study," *Ear and Hearing* 17 (1996): 55–62.

4. Centers for Disease Control and Prevention (CDC), "Summary of 2006 National EHDI Data" (2008). Retrieved on April 22, 2009 from www.cdc gov/ncbddd/ehdi/data.htm; Centers for Disease Control and Prevention (CDC), "Summary of 2011 National EHDI Data" (2013). Retrieved on December 14, 2014 from www.cdc.gov/ncbddd/ehdi/data.htm.

5. Mah-Rya L. Apuzzo and Christine Yoshinaga-Itano, "Early Identification of Infants with Significant Hearing Loss and the Minnesota Child Development Inventory," *Seminars in Hearing* 16 (1995): 124–37; Peter J. Blamey, et al., "Relationships among Speech Perception, Production, Language, Hearing Loss, and Age in Children with Impaired Hearing," *Journal of Speech Language and Hearing Research* 44 (2001): 264–85.

6. Mary Pat Moeller, et al., "Vocalizations of Infants with Hearing Loss Compared with Infants with Normal Hearing: Part I–Phonetic Development," *Ear and Hearing* 28 (2007): 605–27.

7. Patricia K. Kuhl, "A New View of Language Acquisition," *Proceedings of the National Academy of Sciences* 97 (2000): 11850–57; Patricia K. Kuhl, "Speech Perception in Early Infancy: Perceptual Constancy for Spectrally Dissimilar Vowel Categories," *Journal of the Acoustical Society of America* 66 (1979): 1668–79.

8. Christine Yoshinaga-Itano, Diane Coulter, and Vickie Thomson, "The Colorado Newborn Hearing Screening Project: Effects on Speech and Language Development for Children with Hearing Loss," *Journal of Perinatology* 20 (2000): S132–37; Christine Yoshinaga-Itano, et al., "Language of Early- and Later-identified Children with Hearing Loss," *Pediatrics* 102 (1998): 1161–71.

9. Anu Sharma and Julia Campbell, "A Sensitive Period for Cochlear Implantation in Deaf Children," *Journal of Maternal Fetal and Neonatal Medicine* 24 (2011): 151–53.

10. CDC, "Summary of 2011 National EHDI Data" (2013).

11. Kathleen R. Billings and Margaret A. Kenna, "Causes of Pediatric Sensorineural Hearing Loss," *Archives of Otolaryngology Head and Neck Surgery* 125 (1999): 517–21; Josef Shargarodsky et al., "Change in Prevalence of Hearing Loss in US Adolescents," *Journal of the American Medical Association* 304 (2010): 772–78.

12. Janet M. Farrell, "Developing a Strong Early Hearing Detection and Intervention Program," *The ASHA Leader* (March 24, 2009): 8–11; Chia-ling Liu, et al., "Evaluating Loss to Follow-up in Newborn Hearing Screening in Massachusetts," *Pediatrics* 121 (2008): e335–e343.

2. WHAT IS HEARING LOSS?
HOW DID THIS HAPPEN?

1. Fred N. Martin, *Introduction to Audiology*, 6th ed. (Needham Heights, MA: Allyn and Bacon, 1997), 104; Jerry L. Northern and Marion P. Downs, *Hearing in Children*, 5th ed. (Baltimore, Williams & Wilkins, 2002), 67.

2. Northern and Downs, *Hearing in Children*, 45.

3. Allan S. Lieberthal, et al., "The Diagnosis and Management of Acute Otitis Media," *Pediatrics* 131 (2013): e964–99.

4. CDC, "Summary of 2011 national EHDI data" (2013).

5. CDC, "Birth Defects," http://www.cdc.gov/ncbddd/birthdefects/index.html.

6. Joint Committee on Infant Hearing (JCIH), "Year 2007 Position Statement: Principles and Guidelines for Early Hearing Detection and Intervention Programs," *Pediatrics*, 120 (2007): 898–914.

7. David P. Kelsell, et al., "Connexin 26 Mutations in Hereditary Nonsyndromic Sensorineural Hearing Deafness," *Nature* 387 (1997): 80–83; Margaret A. Kenna, et al., "Audiologic Phenotype and Progression in GJB2 (Connexin 26) Hearing Loss," *Archives of Otolaryngology Head and Neck Surgery* 136 (2010): 81–87; and Margaret A. Kenna, et al., "Connexin 26 Studies in Patients with Sensorineural Hearing Loss," *Archives of Otolaryngology Head and Neck Surgery* 127 (2001): 1037–42.

8. Arthur J. Dahle, et al., "Longitudinal Investigation of Hearing Disorders in Children with Congenital Cytomegalovirus," *Journal of the American Academy of Audiology* 11 (2000): 283–90, Karen B. Fowler, et al., "Progressive and Fluctuating Sensorineural Hearing Loss in Children with Asymptomatic Congenital Cytomegalovirus Infection," *Journal of Pediatrics* 130 (1997): 624–30.

9. JCIH, "Year 2007 Position Statement," *Pediatrics*, 120 (2007): 898–914; Brian J. Fligor, "Early Diagnosis and Management of Hearing Loss in Medically Fragile Children," *Seminars in Hearing* 34 (2013): 27–36; Brian J. Fligor and Charlotte H. Mullen, "Audiological Monitoring for Ototoxicity in Medically Complex Children," *Seminars in Hearing* 32 (2011): 273–80.

10. Brian J. Fligor, "Personal Listening Devices and Hearing Loss: Seeking Evidence of a Long-term Problem Through a Successful Short-term Investigation," *Noise and Health* 11 (2009): 129–31; Brian J. Fligor and L. Clarke Cox, "Output Levels of Commercially Available Compact Disc Players and the Potential Risk to Hearing," *Ear and Hearing* 25 (2004): 513–27.

11. Penelope R. Brock, et al., "Platinum-induced Ototoxicity in Children: A Consensus Review on Mechanisms, Predisposition, and Protection, Including a New International Society of Pediatric Oncology Boston Ototoxicity Scale," *Journal of Clinical Oncology* 30 (2012): 2408–17; Brian J. Fligor, et al., "'Accelerated Ear-age' A New Measure of Chemotherapy-induced Ototoxicity," *Pediatric Blood and Cancer* 59 (2012): 947–49; and Kristin Knight, Dale Kraemer, and Edward Neuwalt, "Ototoxicity in Children Receiving Platinum Chemotherapy: Underestimating a Commonly Occurring Toxicity That May Influence

Academic and Social Development," *Journal Clinical Oncology* 23 (2005): 8588–96.

12. U. Ajith Kumar and M. M. Jayaram, "Prevalence and Audiological Characteristics in Individuals with Auditory Neuropathy/Auditory Dys-synchrony," *International Journal of Audiology* 45 (2006): 360–66; Yvonne Sininger and Arnold Starr, *Auditory Neuropathy: A New Perspective on Hearing Disorders* (San Diego, CA: Singular, 2001).

3. HOW HEARING IS TESTED IN INFANTS AND YOUNG CHILDREN

1. JCIH, "Year 2007 Position Statement," *Pediatrics*, 120 (2007): 898–914.

2. "The Marion Downs Center," www.mariondowns.com (accessed December 31, 2014).

3. Jerry L. Northern and Marion P. Downs, *Hearing in Children*, 5th ed. (Baltimore: Williams & Wilkins, 2002), 32.

4. American Academy of Pediatrics, Joint Committee on Infant Hearing, "Joint Committee on Infant Hearing 1994 Position Statement," *Pediatrics* 95 (1995): 152–56.

5. CDC, "Summary of 2011 national EHDI data" (2013).

6. James W. Hall, *New Handbook of Auditory Evoked Responses* (Boston: Pearson, 2007); Kathy R. Vander Werff, Beth A. Prieve, and Lea M. Georgantas, "Infant Air and Bone Conduction Tone Burst Auditory Brain Stem Responses for Classification of Hearing Loss and the Relationship to Behavioral Thresholds," *Ear and Hearing* 30 (2009): 350–68.

7. Sumit Dhar and James W. Hall, *Otoacoustic Emissons: Principles, Procedures, and Protocols* (San Diego, CA: Plural Publishing, 2011).

8. Robert Nozza, "Identification of Otitis Media," in *Children with Hearing Impairment: Contemporary Trends*, ed. Fred H. Bess (Nashville, TN: Vanderbilt Bill Wilkerson Center Press, 1998), 207–14; Robert J. Nozza, et al., "Towards the Validation of Aural Acoustic Immittance Measures for Diagnosis of Middle Ear Effusion in Children," *Ear and Hearing* 13 (1992): 442–53.

4. THE IMPACT OF CHILDHOOD
HEARING LOSS

1. Mary Pat Moeller, "Early Intervention and Language Development in Children Who Are Deaf and Hard of Hearing," *Pediatrics* 106 (2000): 1–9.

2. Julia M. Davis, et al., "Effects of Mild and Moderate Hearing Impairments on Language, Educational, and Psychosocial Behavior of Children," *Journal of Speech and Hearing Disorders* 51 (1986): 53–62.

3. William H. McFarland and F. Blair Simmons, "The Importance of Early Intervention with Severe Childhood Deafness," *Pediatric Annals* 9 (1980): 13–19.

4. Moeller, "Early Intervention and Language Development in Children Who Are Deaf and Hard of Hearing."

5. John B. Brannon and Thomas Murry, "The Spoken Syntax of Normal, Hard-of-Hearing, and Deaf Children," *Journal of Speech and Hearing Research* 9 (1966): 604–10.

6. Ann E. Geers, "Factors Affecting the Development of Speech, Language, and Literacy in Children with Early Cochlear Implantation," *Language Speech and Hearing Services in Schools* 33 (2002): 172–83.

7. Allan S. Lieberthal, et al., "The Diagnosis and Management of Acute Otitis Media."

8. Francis I. Catlin, "Prevention of Hearing Impairment from Infection and Ototoxic Drugs," *Archives of Otolaryngology* 111 (1985): 377–84.

9. Matthew J. Lewis, et al., "Ototoxicity in Children Treated for Osteosarcoma," *Pediatric Blood and Cancer* 52 (2009): 387–91.

10. Patricia Stelmachowicz, et al., "The Importance of High Frequency Audibility in the Speech and Language Development of Children with Hearing Loss," *Archives of Otolaryngology Head and Neck Surgery* 103 (2004): 556–62.

11. Carl C. Crandell and Joseph J. Smaldino, "Classroom Acoustics for Children with Normal Hearing and with Hearing Impairment," *Language Speech and Hearing Services in Schools* 31 (2000): 362–70.

12. Fred H. Bess and Anne Marie Tharpe, "An Introduction to Unilateral Sensorineural Hearing Loss in Children," *Ear and Hearing* 7 (1986): 3–13.

13. Ibid.

5. HOW IS HEARING LOSS TREATED?

1. Lisa S. Davidson and Margaret W. Skinner, "Audibility and Speech Perception of Children Using Wide Dynamic Range Compression Hearing Aids," *American Journal of Audiology* 15 (2006): 141–53.

2. Yvonne S. Sininger, Alison Grimes, and Elizabeth Christensen, "Auditory Development in Early Amplified Children: Factors Influencing Auditory-based Communication Outcomes in Children with Hearing Loss," *Ear and Hearing* 31 (2010): 166–85; Melissa Wake, "Outcomes of Children with Mild-Profound Congenital Hearing Loss at 7 to 8 Years: A Population Study," *Ear and Hearing* 25 (2004): 1–8; and Christine Yoshinaga-Itano, et al., "Language of Early- and Later-identified Children with Hearing Loss," *Pediatrics* 102, no. 5 (1998): 1161–71.

3. BBC News, "Amazing Moment a Deaf Baby Hears for First Time—BBC News." YouTube.com, www.youtube.com/watch?v=T05oyzahoLY (accessed December 31, 2014).

4. American Academy of Audiology (AAA) Clinical Practice Guidelines, "Pediatric Amplification," Reston, VA, 2013, audiology-web.s3.amazonaws.com/migrated/PediatricAmplificationGuide-lines.pdf_539975b3e7e9f1.74471798.pdf (accessed March 1, 2015).

5. Helen E. Cullington and Fan-Gang Zeng, "Speech Recognition with Varying Numbers and Types of Competing Talkers by Normal-hearing, Cochlear-implant, and Implant Simulation Subjects," *Journal of the Acoustical Society of America* 123 (2008): 450–61; Ann E. Geers, "Factors Affecting the Development of Speech, Language, and Literacy in Children with Early Cochlear Implantation," *Language, Speech, and Hearing Services in Schools* 33, no. 3 (2002): 172–83.

6. Arthur Boothroyd, "Auditory Perception of Speech Pattern Contrasts by Subjects with Sensorineural Hearing Loss," *Journal of Speech and Hearing Research* 27 (1984): 134–44.

7. Val Blakely, "Which One Is Deaf?" YouTube.com, www.youtube.com/watch?v=fAtV-DctIeA (accessed February 2, 2015).

8. Cullington and Zeng, "Speech Recognition."

9. Competitiveswimmer, "My Cochlear Implant Activation," YouTube.com, www.youtube.com/watch?v=0B8Zj62LoUg (accessed February 2, 2015).

10. Leah J. Pressman, et al., "Maternal Sensitivity Predicts Language Gain in Preschool Children Who Are Deaf and Hard of Hearing," *Journal of Deaf Studies and Deaf Education* 4 (1999): 294–304.

11. Karen Anderson et al., "Benefit of S/N Enhancing Devices to Speech Perception of Children Listening in a Typical Classroom with Hearing Aids or a Cochlear Implant," *Journal of Educational Audiology* 12 (2005), 14–28.

12. Karen Anderson and Howard Goldstein, "Speech Perception Benefits of FM and Infrared Devices to Children with Hearing Aids in a Typical Classroom," *Language, Speech, and Hearing Services in Schools* 35 (2004): 169–84.

13. MassHAFCC, masshafcc.blogspot.com (accessed January 15, 2015).

14. Brian J. Fligor, "Personal Listening Devices and Hearing Loss: Seeking Evidence of a Long-term Problem Through a Successful Short-term Investigation," *Noise Health* 11, no. 44 (2009): 129–31.

15. Cory D. F. Portnuff, Brian J. Fligor, and Kathryn H. Arehart, "Teenage Use of Portable Listening Devices: A Hazard to Hearing?" *Journal of the American Academy of Audiology* 22 (2011): 663–77.

16. J. Wang, Jean-Luc Puel and R. Bobbin, "Mechanisms of Toxicity in the Cochlea," in *Pharmacology and Ototoxicity for Audiologists*, ed. K. C. M. Campbell (Clifton Park, NY: Thomson Delmar Learning, 2007), 70–85; Alan G. Cheng, et al., "Sensorineural Hearing Loss in Patients with Cystic Fibrosis," *Otolaryngology Head and Neck Surgery* 141 (2009): 86–90; L. H. Bindu and P. P. Reddy, "Genetics of Aminoglycoside Induced and Prelingual Non-syndromic Mitochondrial Hearing Impairment: A Review," *International Journal of Audiology* 47 (2008): 702–07; and Penelope R. Brock, et al., "Platinum-induced Ototoxicity in Children," *Journal of Clinical Oncology* 30, no. 19 (2012): 2408–17.

17. Colleen G. LePrell, "Otoprotective Agents for Prevention of Acquired Hearing Loss in Humans," AudiologyOnline.com, recorded July 31, 2013. www.audiologyonline.com/audiology-ceus/course/otoprotective-agents-for-prevention-acquired-22717.

18. National Institutes of Health, "Early Identification of Hearing Impairment in Infants and Young Children," *NIH Consensus Statement* 11 (1993): 1–24.

19. Brock, et al., "Platinum-induced Ototoxicity in Children."

20. Jonathan I. Matsui and Brenda M. Ryals, "Hair Cell Regeneration: an Exciting Phenomenon . . . But Will Restoring Hearing and Balance Be Possible?" *Journal of Rehabilitation Research and Development* 42 (2005): 187–89.

21. Ibid.

22. Jonathan I. Matsui and Douglas A. Cotanche, "Sensory Hair Cell Death and Regeneration: Two Halves of the Same Equation," *Current Opinion in Otolaryngology Head and Neck Surgery* 12 (2004): 418–25.

23. Jonathan I. Matsui, et al., "Regeneration and Replacement in the Vertebrate Inner Ear," *Drug Discovery Today* 10 (2005): 1307–12.

24. Anu Sharma and Julia Campbell, "A Sensitive Period for Cochlear Implantation," *Journal of Maternal and Fetal Neonatal Medicine* 24 (2011): 151–53.

6. BEYOND DEVICES: HOW DO YOU KNOW INTERVENTIONS ARE WORKING?

1. James E. Mazur, *Learning and Behavior*, 4th ed. (Upper Saddle River, NJ: Prentice Hall, 1998).

2. Suzanne Ducharme, MS, CCC-SLP (Speech-Language Pathologist), personal communication, February 16, 2015.

3. Julia Davis, "Performance of Young Hearing-impaired Children on a Test of Basic Concepts," *Journal of Speech and Hearing Research* 17 (1974): 342–51; Helen M. Robinshaw, "Early Intervention for Hearing Impairment: Differences in the Timing of Communicative and Linguistic Development," *British Journal of Audiology* 29 (1995): 315–34; and Christine Yoshinaga-Itano, et al., "Language of Early- and Later-identified Children with Hearing Loss," *Pediatrics* 102 (1998): 1161–71.

4. Ann Geers and Jean Moog, "Early Speech Perception Test," St. Louis: Central Institute for the Deaf, 1990; Lois L. Elliot and Debra R. Katz, "Development of a New Children's Test of Speech Discrimination," St. Louis: Auditec of St Louis, 1980; and Mark Ross and Jay Lerman, "A Picture Identification Test for Hearing-impaired Children," *Journal of Speech and Hearing Research* 13 (1970): 44–53.

5. Lois L. Elliot and Debra R. Katz, "Children's Pure-tone Detection," *Journal of the Acoustical Society of America* 67 (1980): 343–44; John M. Moore, Wesley R. Wilson, and Gary Thompson, "Visual Reinforcement of Head-turn Responses in Infants under Twelve Months of Age," *Journal of Speech and Hearing Disorders* 42 (1977): 328–34.

6. Karen Anderson, "Early Listening Function (ELF) Instrument for Infants and Toddlers with Hearing Loss," 2002, available from http://successforkidswithhearingloss.com/.

7. Karen Anderson and Joseph Smaldino, "Children's Home Inventory of Listening Difficulties (CHILD)," 2000, available from http://successforkidswithhearingloss.com/.

8. US Department of Education, "Individuals with Disabilities Education Act," http://idea.ed.gov/ (accessed February 4, 2015).

9. American Psychological Association, "Individuals with Disabilities Education Act (IDEA)," http://www.apa.org/about/gr/issues/disability/idea.aspx (accessed February 6, 2015).

10. Better Hearing Institute, "Hearing Loss and Children, in the Classroom," http://www.betterhearing.org/hearing-loss-children/classroom (accessed February 6, 2015).

11. Phonak, "Life Is On," www.phonak.com (accessed February 6, 2015).

12. Oticon, "People First," www.oticon.com (accessed February 6, 2015).

13. Karen Anderson, "Screening Inventory For Targeting Educational Risk (S.I.F.T.E.R.)," 1989, available from http://successforkidswithhearingloss.com; Karen Anderson, "Screening Inventory for Targeting Educational Risk in Secondary Students (Secondary S.I.F.T.E.R.)," 2004, available from http://successforkidswithhearingloss.com.

7. MEMBERS OF THE MANAGEMENT TEAM

1. JCIH, "Supplement to the JCIH 2007 Position Statement," *Pediatrics* March 25, 2013: e1329–e1330, http://pediatrics.aappublications.org/content/early/2013/03/18/peds.2013-0008.citation (accessed April 28, 2013).

2. Ibid., e1330–e1331.

8. EXPERIENCES AND PRACTICAL ADVICE

1. Megan Ford, "Hear My Dreams," http://www.hearmydreams.com (accessed January 7, 2015).

2. Jamie Berke, "Deaf History—Martha's Vineyard," http://deafness.about.com/cs/featurearticles/a/marthasvineyard.htm (accessed February 15, 2015).

3. Bio, "Alexander Graham Bell Biography," http://www.biography.com/people/alexander-graham-bell-9205497 (accessed February 15, 2015).

4. StopBullying.Gov, "Who Is at Risk?" www.stopbullying.gov (accessed February 15, 2015).

5. Ibid, "What Is Bullying?"

6. Michael Squires, et al., "Bullying Is a Safety and Health Issue, How Pediatric Audiologists Can Help," http://www.howsyourhearing.org/documents/bullying.pdf (accessed February 15, 2015).

7. Boston Children's Hospital, "Bullying and Cyberbullying Prevention and Advocacy Collaborative (BACPAC)," http://www.childrenshospital.org/centers-and-services/bullying-and-cyberbullying-prevention-and-advocacy-collaborative-bacpac-program (accessed February 20, 2015).

8. Michael Williams, LICSW, personal communication, June 11, 2011.

BIBLIOGRAPHY

American Academy of Audiology (AAA). "Childhood Hearing Screening Guidelines." Reston, VA. 2011. Accessed February 15, 2015 from www.audiology.org/resources/documentlibrary/Documents/ChildhoodScreeningGuidelines.pdf.

American Academy of Audiology (AAA) Clinical Practice Guidelines. "Pediatric Amplification." Reston, VA. 2013. Accessed March 1, 2015 from audiology-web.s3.amazonaws.com/migrated/PediatricAmplificationGuidelines.pdf_539975b3e7e9f1.74471798.pdf.

American Academy of Pediatrics, Joint Committee on Infant Hearing. "Joint Committee on Infant Hearing 1994 Position Statement." *Pediatrics* 95 (1995): 152–56.

———. "Year 2000 Position Statement: Principles and Guidelines for Early Hearing Detection and Intervention Programs." *American Journal of Audiology* 9 (2000): 9–29.

American Psychological Association. "Individuals with Disabilities Education Act (IDEA)." Accessed February 6, 2015 from http://www.apa.org/about/gr/issues/disability/idea.aspx.

Anderson, Karen. "Screening Inventory For Targeting Educational Risk (S.I.F.T.E.R.)." (1989). Available from http://successforkidswithhearingloss.com/.

———. "Early Listening Function (ELF) Instrument for Infants and Toddlers with Hearing Loss." (2002). Available from http://successforkidswithhearingloss.com/.

———. "Screening Inventory For Targeting Educational Risk in Secondary Students (Secondary S.I.F.T.E.R.)." 2004. Available from http://successforkidswithhearingloss.com/.

Anderson, Karen, et al. "Benefit of S/N Enhancing Devices to Speech Perception of Children Listening in a Typical Classroom with Hearing Aids or a Cochlear Implant." *Journal of Educational Audiology* 12 (2005): 14–28.

Anderson, Karen, and Howard Goldstein. "Speech Perception Benefits of FM and Infrared Devices to Children with Hearing Aids in a Typical Classroom." *Language, Speech, and Hearing Services in Schools* 35 (2004): 169–84.

Anderson, Karen, and Joseph Smaldino. "Children's Home Inventory of Listening Difficulties (CHILD)." (2000). Available from http://successforkidswithhearingloss.com/.

Apuzzo, Mah-Rya L., and Christine Yoshinaga-Itano. "Early Identification of Infants with Significant Hearing Loss and the Minnesota Child Development Inventory." *Seminars in Hearing* 16 (1995): 124–37.

BBC News. "Amazing Moment a Deaf Baby Hears for First Time—BBC News." You-Tube.com. Accessed December 31, 2014 from www.youtube.com/watch?v=T05oyzahoLY.

Berke, Jamie. "Deaf History—Martha's Vineyard." Accessed February 15, 2015 from http://deafness.about.com/cs/featurearticles/a/marthasvineyard.htm.

Bess, Fred H., and Jack L. Paradise. "Universal Screening for Infant Hearing Impairment: Not Simple, Not Risk Free, Not Necessarily Beneficial, and Not Presently Justified." *Pediatrics* 93 (1994): 330–34.

Bess, Fred H., and Anne Marie Tharpe. "An Introduction to Unilateral Sensorineural Hearing Loss in Children." *Ear and Hearing* 7 (1986): 3–13.

Better Hearing Institute. "Hearing Loss and Children, in the Classroom." Accessed February 6, 2015 fromhttp://www.betterhearing.org/hearing-loss-children/classroom.

Billings, Kathleen R., and Margaret A. Kenna. "Causes of Pediatric Sensorineural Hearing Loss." *Archives of Otolaryngology Head and Neck Surgery* 125 (1999): 517–21.

Bindu, L. H., and P. P. Reddy. "Genetics of Aminoglycoside Induced and Prelingual Non-syndromic Mitochondrial Hearing Impairment: A Review." *International Journal of Audiology* 47 (2008): 702–7.

Bio. "Alexander Graham Bell Biography." Accessed February 15, 2015 from http://www.biography.com/people/alexander-graham-bell-9205497.

Blakely, Val. "Which One Is Deaf?" YouTube.com. Accessed February 2, 2015 from www.youtube.com/watch?v=fAtV-DctIeA.

Blamey, Peter J., et al. "Relationships Among Speech Perception, Production, Language, Hearing Loss, and Age in Children with Impaired Hearing." *Journal of Speech Language and Hearing Research* 44 (2001): 264–85.

Boothroyd, Arthur. "Auditory Perception of Speech Pattern Contrasts by Subjects with Sensorineural Hearing Loss." *Journal of Speech and Hearing Research* 27 (1984): 134–44.

Boston Children's Hospital. "Bullying and Cyberbullying Prevention and Advocacy Collaborative (BACPAC)." Accessed February 20, 2015 from http://www.childrenshospital.org/centers-and-services/bullying-and-cyberbullying-prevention-and-advocacy-collaborative-bacpac-program.

Brannon, John B., and Thomas Murry. "The Spoken Syntax of Normal, Hard-of-Hearing, and Deaf Children." *Journal of Speech and Hearing Research* 9 (1966): 604–10.

Brock, Penelope R., et al. "Platinum-induced Ototoxicity in Children: A Consensus Review on Mechanisms, Predisposition, and Protection, Including a New International Society of Pediatric Oncology Boston Ototoxicity Scale." *Journal of Clinical Oncology* 30 (2012): 2408–17.

Catlin, Francis I. "Prevention of Hearing Impairment from Infection and Ototoxic Drugs." *Archives of Otolaryngology* 111 (1985): 377–84.

Centers for Disease Control and Prevention (CDC). Summary of 2006 National EHDI Data. (2008). Retrieved on April 22, 2009 from www.cdc.gov/ncbddd/ehdi/data.htm.

———. Summary of 2011 National EHDI Data. (2013). Retrieved on December 14, 2014 from www.cdc.gov/ncbddd/ehdi/data.htm.

———. Birth Defects. Retrieved on December 14, 2014 from http://www.cdc.gov/ncbddd/birthdefects/index.html.

Chang, Kay W., et al. "External and Middle Ear Status Related to Evoked Otoacoustic Emission in Neonates." *Archives of Otolaryngology Head and Neck Surgery* 119 (1993): 276–83.

Cheng, Alan G., et al. "Sensorineural Hearing Loss in Patients with Cystic Fibrosis." *Otolaryngology Head and Neck Surgery* 141 (2009): 86–90.

Competitive swimmer. "My Cochlear Implant Activation." YouTube.com. Accessed February 2, 2015 from www.youtube.com/watch?v=0B8Zj62LoUg.

Cox, L. Clarke. "Infant Assessment: Developmental and Age-related Considerations." In Jacobson, J. T., ed. *The Auditory Brainstem Response*, 297–316. San Diego, CA: College Hill Press, 1985.

Crandell, Carl C., and Joseph J. Smaldino. "Classroom Acoustics for Children with Normal Hearing and with Hearing Impairment." *Language Speech and Hearing Services in Schools* 31 (2000): 362–70.

Cullington, Helen E., and Fan-Gang Zeng. "Speech Recognition with Varying Numbers and Types of Competing Talkers by Normal-hearing, Cochlear-implant, and Implant Simulation Subjects." *Journal of the Acoustical Society of America* 123 (2008): 450–61.

Dahle, Arthur J., et al. "Longitudinal Investigation of Hearing Disorders in Children with Congenital Cytomegalovirus." *Journal of the American Academy of Audiology* 11 (2000): 283–90.

Davidson, Lisa S., and Margaret W. Skinner. "Audibility and Speech Perception of Children Using Wide Dynamic Range Compression Hearing Aids." *American Journal of Audiology* 15 (2006): 141–53.

Davis, Julia. "Performance of Young Hearing-impaired Children on a Test of Basic Concepts." *Journal of Speech and Hearing Research* 17 (1974): 342–51.

Davis, Julia M., et al. "Effects of Mild and Moderate Hearing Impairments on Language, Educational, and Psychosocial Behavior of Children." *Journal of Speech and Hearing Disorders* 51 (1986): 53–62.

Dhar, Sumit, and James W. Hall. *Otoacoustic Emissons: Principles, Procedures, and Protocols.* San Diego, CA: Plural Publishing, 2011.

Dornan, Briana, et al. "Pediatric Hearing Assessment by Auditory Brainstem Response in the Operating Room." *International Journal of Pediatric Otorhinolaryngology* 75 (2011): 935–38.

Elliot, Lois L., and Debra R. Katz. "Children's Pure-tone Detection." *Journal of the Acoustical Society of America* 67 (1980): 343–44.

———. "Development of a New Children's Test of Speech Discrimination." St. Louis: Auditec of St. Louis, 1980.

Farrell, Janet M. "Developing a Strong Early Hearing Detection and Intervention Program." *The ASHA Leader* (March 24, 2009). 8–11.

Fligor, Brian J. "Personal Listening Devices and Hearing Loss: Seeking Evidence of a Long Term Problem Through a Successful Short-term Investigation." *Noise and Health* 11(2009): 129–31.

———. "Early Diagnosis and Management of Hearing Loss in Medically Fragile Children." *Seminars in Hearing* 34 (2013): 27–36.

Fligor, Brian J., and L. Clarke Cox. "Output Levels of Commercially Available Compact Disc Players and the Potential Risk to Hearing." *Ear and Hearing* 25 (2004): 513–27.

Fligor, Brian J., et al. "Factors Associated with Sensorineural Hearing Loss in Survivors of Extracorporeal Membrane Oxygenation Therapy." *Pediatrics* 115 (2005): 1519–28.

Fligor, Brian J., et al. "'Accelerated Ear-age' A New Measure of Chemotherapy-induced Ototoxicity." *Pediatric Blood and Cancer* 59 (2012): 947–49.

Fligor, Brian J., Sandra Levey, and Tania Levey. "Cultural and Demographic Factors Influencing Noise Exposure Estimates from Use of Portable Listening Devices in an Urban Environment." *Journal of Speech Language and Hearing Research* 57 (2014): 1535–47.

Fligor, Brian J., and Charlotte H. Mullen. "Audiological Monitoring for Ototoxicity in Medically Complex Children." *Seminars in Hearing* 32 (2011): 273–80.

Ford, Megan. "Hear My Dreams." Accessed January 7, 2015 from http://www.hearmydreams.com.

Fowler, Karen B., et al. "Progressive and Fluctuating Sensorineural Hearing Loss in Children with Asymptomatic Congenital Cytomegalovirus Infection." *Journal of Pediatrics* 130 (1997): 624–30.

Geers, Ann E. "Factors Affecting the Development of Speech, Language, and Literacy in Children with Early Cochlear Implantation." *Language Speech and Hearing Services in Schools* 33 (2002): 172–83.

Geers, Ann, and Jean Moog. "Factors Predictive of the Development of Literacy in Profoundly Hearing-impaired Adolescents." *Volta Review* 91 (1989): 69–86.

———. "Early Speech Perception Test." St. Louis: Central Institute for the Deaf, 1990.

Gorga, Michael P., et al. "Some Issues Relevant to Establishing a Universal Newborn Hearing Screening Program." *Journal of the American Academy of Audiology* 12 (2001): 101–12.

Gravel, Judith, et al. "New York State Universal Newborn Hearing Screening Demonstration Project: Effects of Screening Protocol on Inpatient Outcome Measures." *Ear and Hearing* 21 (2000): 131–40.

Hall, James W. *New Handbook of Auditory Evoked Responses*. Boston: Pearson, 2007.

Harrison, Melody, and Jackson Roush. "Age of Suspicion, Identification, and Intervention for Infants and Young Children with Hearing Loss: A National Study." *Ear and Hearing* 17 (1996): 55–62.

Joint Committee on Infant Hearing (JCIH). "Year 2007 Position Statement: Principles and Guidelines for Early Hearing Detection and Intervention Programs." *Pediatrics*, 120 (2007): 898–914.

———. "Supplement to the JCIH 2007 Position Statement: Principles and Guidelines for Early Intervention After Confirmation That a Child Is Deaf or Hard of Hearing." *Pediatrics* March 25, 2013: e1324–e1349, http://pediatrics.aappublications.org/content/early/2013/03/18/peds.2013-0008.citation.

Kelsell, David P., et al. "Connexin 26 Mutations in Hereditary Non-syndromic Sensorineural Hearing Deafness." *Nature* 387 (1997): 80–83.

Kenna, Margaret A., et al. "Connexin 26 Studies in Patients with Sensorineural Hearing Loss." *Archives of Otolaryngology Head and Neck Surgery* 127 (2001): 1037–42.

Kenna, Margaret A., et al. "Audiologic Phenotype and Progression in GJB2 (Connexin 26) Hearing Loss." *Archives of Otolaryngology Head and Neck Surgery* 136 (2010): 81–87.

Kennedy, Colin R., et al. "Language Ability after Early Detection of Permanent Childhood Hearing Impairment." *New England Journal of Medicine* 354 (2006): 2131–41.

Kingsley, Emily Pearl. "Welcome to Holland," *www.our-kids.org*. 1987.http://www.our-kids.org/Archives/Holland.html.

Knight, Kristin, Dale Kraemer, and Edward Neuwalt. "Ototoxity in Children Receiving Platinum Chemotherapy: Underestimating a Commonly Occurring Toxicity That May Influence Academic and Social Development." *Journal Clinical Oncology* 23 (2005): 8588–96.

Kuhl, Patricia K. "Speech Perception in Early Infancy: Perceptual Constancy for Spectrally Dissimilar Vowel Categories." *Journal of the Acoustical Society of America* 66 (1979): 1668–79.

———. "A New View of Language Acquisition." *Proceedings of the National Academy of Sciences* 97 (2000): 11850–57.

Kumar, U. Ajith, and M. M. Jayaram. "Prevalence and Audiological Characteristics in Individuals with Auditory Neuropathy/Auditory Dys-synchrony." *International Journal of Audiology* 45 (2006): 360–66.

LePrell, Colleen G. "Otoprotective Agents for Prevention of Acquired Hearing Loss in Humans." AudiologyOnline.com. Recorded July 31, 2013.www.audiologyonline.com/audiology-ceus/course/otoprotective-agents-for-prevention-acquired-22717.

Levey, Sandra, Tania Levey, and Brian J. Fligor. "Noise Exposure Estimates of Urban MP3 Player Users." *Journal of Speech Language and Hearing Research* 54 (2011): 263–77.

Lewis, Matthew J., et al. "Ototoxicity in Children Treated for Osteosarcoma." *Pediatric Blood and Cancer* 52 (2009): 387–91.

Lieberthal, Allan S., et al. "The Diagnosis and Management of Acute Otitis Media." *Pediatrics* 131 (2013): e964–99.

Liu, Chia-ling., et al. "Evaluating Loss to Follow-up in Newborn Hearing Screening in Massachusetts." *Pediatrics* 121 (2008): e335–e343.

Marion Downs Center, The.www.mariondowns.com. Accessed December 31, 2014.

Martin, Fred N. *Introduction to Audiology*, 6th ed. Needham Heights, MA: Allyn and Bacon, 1997.

MassHAFCC. masshafcc.blogspot.com. Accessed January 15, 2015.

Matsui, Jonathan I., and Douglas A. Cotanche. "Sensory Hair Cell Death and Regeneration: Two Halves of the Same Equation. *Current Opinion in Otolaryngology Head and Neck Surgery* 12 (2004): 418–25.

Matsui, Jonathan I., et al. "Regeneration and Replacement in the Vertebrate Inner Ear." *Drug Discovery Today* 10 (2005): 1307–12.

Matsui, Jonathan I., and Brenda M. Ryals. "Hair Cell Regeneration: An Exciting Phenomenon . . . But Will Restoring Hearing and Balance Be Possible?" *Journal of Rehabilitation Research and Development* 42 (2005): 187–89.

Mazur, James E. *Learning and Behavior*, 4th ed. Upper Saddle River, NJ: Prentice Hall, 1998

McFarland, William H., and F. Blair Simmons. "The Importance of Early Intervention with Severe Childhood Deafness." *Pediatric Annals* 9 (1980): 13–19.

Moeller, Mary Pat. "Early Intervention and Language Development in Children Who are Deaf and Hard of Hearing." *Pediatrics* 106 (2000): 1–9.

Moeller, Mary Pat, et al. "Vocalizations of Infants with Hearing Loss Compared with Infants with Normal Hearing: Part I–Phonetic Development." *Ear and Hearing* 28 (2007): 605–27.

Moeller, Mary Pat, Karl R. White, and Lenore Shisler. "Primary Care Physicians' Knowledge, Attitudes, and Practices Related to Newborn Hearing Screening." *Pediatrics* 118 (2006): 1357–70.

Moore, John M., Wesley R. Wilson, and Gary Thompson. "Visual Reinforcement of Head-turn Responses in Infants under Twelve Months of Age." *Journal of Speech and Hearing Disorders* 42 (1977): 328–34.

National Institutes of Health. "Early Identification of Hearing Impairment in Infants and Young Children." *NIH Consensus Statement* 11 (1993): 1–24.

Northern, Jerry L., and Marion P. Downs. *Hearing in Children*, 5th ed. Baltimore: Williams & Wilkins, 2002.

Norton, Susan J., et al. "Identification of Neonatal Hearing Impairment: Evaluation of TE-OAE, DPOAE, and ABR Test Performance." *Ear and Hearing* 21 (2000): 508–28.

Nozza Robert. "Identification of Otitis Media." In Bess, F., ed. *Children with Hearing Impairment: Contemporary Trends*, 207–14. Nashville, TN: Vanderbilt Bill Wilkerson Center Press, 1998.

Nozza, Robert J., et al. "Towards the Validation of Aural Acoustic Immittance Measures for Diagnosis of Middle Ear Effusion in Children." *Ear and Hearing* 13 (1992): 442–53.

Oticon. "People First." Accessed February 6, 2015 from www.oticon.com.

Phonak. "Life Is On." Accessed February 6, 2015 from www.phonak.com.

Portnuff, Cory D. F., Brian J. Fligor, Kathryn H. Arehart. "Teenage Use of Portable Listening Devices: A Hazard to Hearing?" *Journal of the American Academy of Audiology* 22 (2011): 663–77.

———. "Self-report and Long-term Field Measures of MP3 Player Use: How Accurate Is Self-report?" *International Journal of Audiology* 52 Suppl. 1 (2013): S33–40.

Pressman, Leah J., et al. "Maternal Sensitivity Predicts Language Gain in Preschool Children Who Are Deaf and Hard of Hearing." *Journal of Deaf Studies and Deaf Education* 4 (1999): 294–304.

Robinshaw, Helen M. "Early Intervention for Hearing Impairment: Differences in the Timing of Communicative and Linguistic Development." *British Journal of Audiology* 29 (1995): 315–34.

Ross, Mark, and Jay Lerman. "A Picture Identification Test for Hearing-impaired Children." *Journal of Speech and Hearing Research* 13 (1970): 44–53.

Shargarordsky, Josef, et al. "Change in Prevalence of Hearing Loss in US Adolescents." *Journal of the American Medical Association* 304 (2010): 77–78.

Sharma, Anu, and Julia Campbell. "A Sensitive Period for Cochlear Implantation in Deaf Children." *Journal of Maternal-Fetal and Neonatal Medicine* 24 (2011): 151–53.

Shepard, Neil, et al. "Characteristics of Hearing-impaired Children in the Public Schools: Part I—Demographic Data." *Journal of Speech and Hearing Disorders* 46 (1981): 123–29.

Sininger, Yvonne S., et al. "Newborn Hearing Screening Speeds Diagnosis and Access to Intervention By 20–25 Months." *Journal of the American Academy of Audiology* 20 (2009): 49–57.

Sininger, Yvonne S., Alison Grimes, and Elizabeth Christensen. "Auditory Development in Early Amplified Children: Factors Influencing Auditory-based Communication Outcomes in Children with Hearing Loss." *Ear and Hearing* 31 (2010): 166–85.

Sininger, Yvonne, and Arnold Starr. *Auditory Neuropathy: A New Perspective on Hearing Disorders*. San Diego, CA: Singular, 2001.

Squires, Michael, et al. "Bullying Is a Safety and Health Issue, How Pediatric Audiologists Can Help." *AudiologyToday* Sept/Oct (2013): 18–26. Accessed February 15, 2015 from http://www.howsyourhearing.org/documents/bullying.pdf.

Stapells, David R., and Peggy Oates. "Estimation of the Pure Tone Audiogram by the Auditory Brainstem Response: A Review." *Audiology and Neurotology* 2 (1997): 257–80.

Stelmachowicz, Patricia, et al. "The Importance of High Frequency Audibility in the Speech and Language Development of Children with Hearing Loss." *Archives of Otolaryngology Head and Neck Surgery* 103 (2004): 556–62.

Stickney, Ginger S., et al. "Cochlear Implant Speech Recognition with Speech Maskers." *Journal of the Acoustical Society of America* 116 (2004): 1081–91.

StopBullying.Gov. "Who Is at Risk?" Accessed February 15, 2015 from www.stopbullying.gov.

US Department of Education. "Individuals with Disabilities Education Act." Accessed February 4, 2015 from http://idea.ed.gov/.

Vander Werff, Kathy R., Beth A. Prieve, and Lea M. Georgantas. "Infant Air and Bone Conduction Tone Burst Auditory Brain Stem Responses for Classification of Hearing Loss and the Relationship to Behavioral Thresholds." *Ear and Hearing* 30 (2009): 350–68.

Vohr, Betty R., et al. "The Rhode Island Hearing Assessment Program: Experience with Statewide Hearing Screening (1993–1996)." *The Journal of Pediatrics* 133 (1998): 353–57.

Wake, Melissa. "Outcomes of Children with Mild-Profound Congenital Hearing Loss at 7 to 8 Years: A Population Study." *Ear and Hearing* 25 (2004): 1–8.

Wang J., Jean-Luc Puel, and Bobbin R. "Mechanisms of Toxicity in the Cochlea." In Campbell K. C. M., ed. *Pharmacology and Ototoxicity for Audiologists*, 70–85. Clifton Park, NY: Thomson Delmar Learning, 2007.

Yoshinaga-Itano, Christine, Diane Coulter, and Vickie Thomson. "The Colorado Newborn Hearing Screening Project: Effects on Speech and Language Development for Children with Hearing Loss." *Journal of Perinatology* 20 (2000): S132–37.

Yoshinaga-Itano, Christine, et al. "Language of Early- and Later-identified Children with Hearing Loss." *Pediatrics* 102 (1998): 1161–71.

INDEX

ABOUT THE AUTHOR

Brian J. Fligor is an audiologist, engineer, musician, and avid music enthusiast. He received a BS in biomedical engineering in 1997 and ScD in audiology in 2002, both degrees from Boston University. He completed his clinical fellowship in audiology in 2002 at Boston Children's Hospital and a postdoctoral fellowship at Boston Children's Hospital/Harvard Medical School in 2004. He was director of diagnostic audiology at Boston Children's Hospital and clinical faculty at Harvard Medical School 2005–2013. He is a graduate, and subsequently faculty, of the Boston Children's Hospital Leadership Education in Neurodevelopmental and Related Disabilities. Currently, Dr. Fligor is chief audiology officer at Lantos Technologies, a private Boston-area medical device company developing novel technology to treat and prevent hearing loss. He maintains a private practice, Boston Audiology Consultants, focused on audiological care of children and musicians.

Dr. Fligor's dissertation on potential risk for hearing loss from using portable listening devices/headphones was published in 2004, which precipitated a firestorm of scientific debate and popular media coverage about hearing loss risk from using iPods/MP3 players. His research was spoofed in a skit on The Late Show with David Letterman in 2005. Dr. Fligor's clinical practice and research into childhood hearing loss caused by aggressive medical interventions has been incorporated into best-practice guidelines promoted by the Joint Committee on Infant

Hearing and the Children's Oncology Group. He is a member of a technical advisory committee to the World Health Organization on thoughtful approaches to effectively mitigate risk for hearing loss from headphones. He lives in the metropolitan Boston area with his wife and four children.